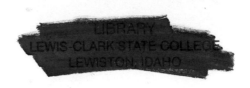
Dying and Living in the Neighborhood

DYING and LIVING in the NEIGHBORHOOD

A Street-Level View of America's Healthcare Promise

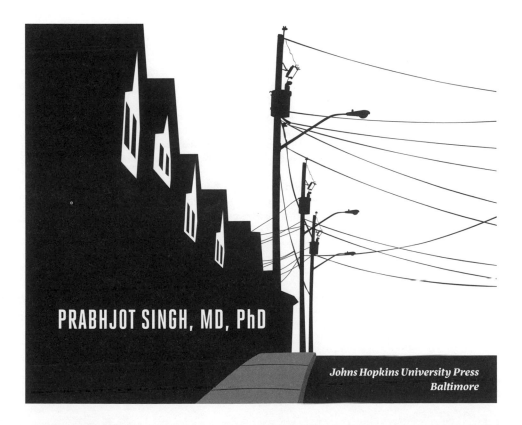

PRABHJOT SINGH, MD, PhD

Johns Hopkins University Press
Baltimore

Johns Hopkins University Press
2715 North Charles Street
Baltimore, Maryland 21218-4363
www.press.jhu.edu

Library of Congress Cataloging-in-Publication Data

Names: Singh, Prabhjot, 1982– , author.
Title: Dying and living in the neighborhood : a street-level view of America's healthcare
    promise / Prabhjot Singh.
Description: Baltimore : Johns Hopkins University Press, 2016. | Includes bibliographical
    references and index.
Identifiers: LCCN 2015046696 | ISBN 9781421420448 (hardcover : alk. paper) |
    ISBN 1421420449 (hardcover : alk. paper) | ISBN 9781421420455 (electronic) |
    ISBN 1421420457 (electronic)
Subjects: MESH: Community Health Services | Preventive Health Services |
    Health Promotion | Health Policy | Chronic Disease—prevention & control |
    Socioeconomic Factors | United States | Systems Architecting & Engineering |
Classification: LCC RA418 | NLM WA 546 AA1 | DDC 362.1—dc23
    LC record available at http://lccn.loc.gov/2015046696

A catalog record for this book is available from the British Library.

*Special discounts are available for bulk purchases of this book. For more information, please contact
Special Sales at 410-516-6936 or specialsales@press.jhu.edu.*

Johns Hopkins University Press uses environmentally friendly book materials, including
recycled text paper that is composed of at least 30 percent post-consumer waste, whenever
possible.

O physician, you are a competent physician, if you first diagnose the disease.
Prescribe such a remedy, by which all sorts of illnesses may be cured.
—Guru Nanak (d. 1469 CE)

Contents

Preface

If this man is a physician . . . then it is self-evident that his science must include whatever is pertinent to his proclaimed purpose.
—Rudolph Virchow, 1848

In 1982, the year I was born, the historian John Burnham wrote an article in *Science* entitled, "American Medicine's Golden Age: What Happened to It?"[1] This was the same year as the Chicago murders involving poisoned Tylenol capsules, which heightened a sense of danger in one of our most trusted industries, and the same year that Medicare began to fund hospice care. In the years since Burnham's article, scientific innovation like the Human Genome Project and healthcare management inventions like the health maintenance organization were both oversold to the American public as immediately advancing our ability to live healthier lives. I started medical and graduate school 20 years later, amidst rapidly rising healthcare costs, horror stories about hospital errors, a stagnant national biomedical research budget, and more than 40 million uninsured Americans. My colleagues and I inherited a narrative of healthcare in deep crisis, told by a profession hovering around its nadir.

In 2014, my last year of internal medicine residency, cardiologist Sandeep Jauhar published a widely read memoir entitled *Doctored: The Disillusionment of an American Physician*. He reported that only 6 percent of physicians had positive morale.[2] My own path to clinical practice included graduate work as part of the National Institutes of Health's Medical Scientist Training Program, which I undertook at Weill Cornell Medical College and Rockefeller University, where I grew interested in systems analysis, networks, and information theory. This combined training was meant to bring together the best of both clinical and scientific training and culture. My cohort of physician-scientists was charged with leading the nation in "translational science," which would form a bridge between the laboratory bench and the bedside. But even at Rockefeller, which is recognized as an epicenter of major scientific advances (and home to four Nobel Prize winners in the five years before I began my training), there was a similar malaise. We heard rising and established professors lament the state of biomedical research, which was increasingly perceived as an insider game of grant writing in an overly competitive funding environment. Scientists and physicians alike were (and are) upset that they could not simply do what they were trained to do. Instead, paperwork dominated the time of both, pushing the work of research and patient care to the margins.

This chastening has happened fairly quickly for an old and intense profession. My twenty-first-century training as a physician-scientist had a charming mid-twentieth-century flavor to it, lovingly shaped by people who were paragons of caring physicians and brilliant scientists. My colleagues and I spent years in small rooms, staring down the barrel of microscopes or moving precise aliquots of biological components with pipettes, or examining the skin and organs of patients and learning how to successfully draw blood. We communicated as peers within tight networks of researchers and from the bottom of strict hospital hierarchies.

If anything, our training took us back in time to the dawn of modern medical schools in 1910, when Abraham Flexner (backed by the Carnegie Foundation's checkbook) took a strong stance in support of scientific medicine and against "alternatives" (e.g., naturopathic, homeopathic, osteopathic, chiropractic medicine). The first two years of medical school seemed to be designed to reinforce the supremacy of biomedicine over quackery, while the last two clinical years taught us how to apply the findings of biomedical and clinical research to the treatment of the patients in front of us. The most visible signs of a modern age were in the devices around us rather than in the methods we used to construct a differential diagnosis, devise a plan, and then communicate both to the patient in question.

By the time I started my graduate work at Rockefeller, under an extraordinarily kind scientist in the area of neural and genetic systems, I felt constrained by the kinds of questions that medical and scientific culture seemed reluctant to answer. Certainly, not all of my peers felt this way, and the brilliant and persistent among them found creative ways to move forward. But like thousands of others across the country, I looked abroad, to the poorest countries in the world and the growing field of global health, to find promise and purpose. I gravitated toward sub-Saharan Africa, where my parents were born and where I spent my early childhood before moving to Michigan and Pennsylvania, and finally, New York City.

•   •   •

Despite the limited resources, technology, and infrastructure, the opportunities I had alongside my experiences abroad were extraordinary. I joined the International Rescue Committee to learn about global population health in the context of refugee camps across the world. Because of my scientific background, they thought I could build an information system that would help them monitor the needs of thousands of refugees and anticipate the necessary supplies before they ran out. There was little in my medical training that prepared me for this task, except for the confidence to try. I built what they needed, which enabled them to demonstrate that a dynamic feedback system was as critically necessary as the needs and supplies it tracked. I predominantly spent time within sub-Saharan Africa, where I had the chance to see—through a different, analytical lens—the places where my family had lived since moving from the Punjab at the turn of the twentieth century.

Throughout my travels, I thought about another nineteenth-century phenomenon: the work of Rudolph Virchow, German physician, anthropologist, politician, and scientist, whom I had learned about from my college history professor, Theodore Brown. Virchow is credited with bringing scientific thought to medicine, linking economic and political development with health improvement, and advancing the social dimensions of public health. Virchow provided me with a sharpened view of what medicine should be, one that implies a different culture of medicine than what prevails today. "Medicine is a social science, and politics is nothing else but medicine on a large scale. Medicine, as a social science, as the science of human beings, has the obligation to point out problems and to attempt their theoretical solution: the politician, the practical anthropologist, must find the means for their actual solution."[3]

In a translation that Brown co-authored, I was surprised by Virchow's views on how to address a devastating outbreak of typhus in a poor rural area of Prussia, where "ethnic Poles" lived under the thumb of empire. Without suggesting that scientific inquiry and clinical services were less important, he recognized that social, economic, and political reform came hand in hand with achieving better health. He saw that better health and socioeconomic development are intertwined and that healthcare at its best is a feedback loop that potentiates both:

If we therefore wish to intervene in Upper Silesia, we must begin to promote
the advancement of the entire population, and to stimulate a common general effort. A population will never achieve full education, freedom and prosperity in the form of a gift from the outside. The people must acquire what
they need by their own efforts [...] Therefore, I abide by the doctrine which
I have placed at the head of this discussion: *Free and unlimited democracy.*[4]

For Virchow, in the physician's role as the "natural attorney for the poor,"
the domain of the physician crossed over into politics when politics failed
the people. He was declared a radical for recommending the "introduction
of Polish as an official language, democratic self-government, separation of
church and state, and the creation of grassroots agricultural cooperatives."[5]

As I traveled in East and West Africa to refugee encampments that
seemed as marginalized as Virchow's "ethnic Poles," I had no idea how his
inspiring ideas might be reconciled with my education to date, except that
the demands of my work there echoed his themes. We had a new armament
of effective therapies for malaria, pneumonia, diarrhea, tuberculosis, para-
sites, and AIDS, but without the infrastructure to deliver them, the work of
designing a basic healthcare system would have to be intertwined with the
political and economic advancement of a region.

As I was finishing my PhD, I took a leave to pursue a postdoctoral fellowship in sustainable development with the macroeconomist Jeffrey Sachs
and pediatrician Sonia Sachs at Columbia University, within an integrated
rural development project called the Millennium Villages Project (MVP).
I was drawn to this work because it sought to break a cycle of poverty from
the inside out, connecting ten different sites in a network in which they
could learn from each other as they found their way—and in which the
broader, external community of experts and advocates could trade insights
as their various forms of expertise and resources were called upon.

My specific role was to develop a community health worker (CHW)
subsystem that would enable locally hired and rapidly trained lay community members to serve as links between clinics and their communities.
They would have paid, full-time jobs, mobile phones, a graduated path to
professional advancement, and training in point-of-care diagnostics and
therapies. Without a functioning CHW subsystem, children died of preventable illness before reaching the clinic and families had as many children as
possible in anticipation of their potential loss. This left families poorer and

undersupplied when most children survived and they had more mouths to feed, exposing kids and adults to malnutrition and illness. Survival was rewarded with ever-dividing inheritances of increasingly small parcels of land, far away from robust markets and industry where one could earn a living wage. This meant that kids were pulled from school to find work, leading to uneducated adults and forestalling any chance of regional economic development, this last being a precondition for greater investments in healthcare systems. That's the theory, anyway, one that is exceedingly hard to test.

Figuring out how to build a CHW subsystem of the healthcare system allowed me to put some of my scientific training in systems analysis to use, all while learning about public health and economic development. For the most part, I learned by doing, taking cues from regional experts along with existing CHWs and the communities they served. My job was to learn how places across the world—from Brazil to Ethiopia to India—had built these subsystems and to transfer those lessons to regionally hired managers in the ten MVP sites. Then I worked with the villages to build appropriate feedback loops between the community, CHW subsystem, and overarching healthcare system so they could independently figure out what was and was not working. After that, my team was in learning-and-sharing mode, until the entire effort was shifted to regional centers in East and West Africa. Occasionally, a technological development, like the rise of mobile phones or a new rapid diagnostic test for malaria, led us to reengage and facilitate redesign where necessary.

Along the way, there were specific policy barriers that posed a significant challenge to the functioning of the community health worker systems. In some countries, it was illegal to pay these workers. In others, they were not permitted to do certain activities. In order to address these issues, it was important to work with the government, relevant business and industry, community advocates, and a raft of nongovernmental organizations to find the right time and place (e.g., local, state, or federal) to see how a new approach might work.

The greatest challenge was co-designing a healthcare system with the work, ideas, and investment of community members in the broader context of co-designing education and agricultural and food distribution systems while fostering small business development—which all engage the same community members. I say co-designing because in addition to community members, other parties included development experts, public health practitioners, business owners, and local and national politicians, all of whom have goals of their own. Since Virchow's time, this project has been pursued in various forms. Sachs argues,[6] persuasively, that the MVP efforts are distinguished by an unprecedented constellation of factors: advances in technology (medication, diagnostic devices, mobile phones), large-scale linkages between health improvement and national economic development, and the integration of multiple public sectors (education, agriculture, small business development, infrastructure). Most people would agree that these components are well known, but the kinds of systems that emerge when a *community* puts it all together are what the multicountry learning network was working to figure out. In 2016, the MVP publishes its summative findings. In the meantime, it has become clear to me that the everything-at-once method can be as overwhelming as the test-things-one-by-one method can be insufficient. Perhaps most importantly, I learned firsthand that the people who have to live with the uncertain consequences of socioeconomic decisions ought to play a significant role in defining their purpose.

When I returned from my leave of absence to finish my final year of medical school at New York Hospital in 2011, the Patient Protection and Affordable Care Act (ACA), President Obama's signature health legislation, was beginning to make its presence felt outside of Washington. I began the jarring process of figuring out how the revelations of MVP's work in rural sub-Saharan Africa might be translated to American healthcare. It is not far-fetched to presume that low-income, resource-constrained settings have their correlatives in America. Many of our nation's neighborhoods have life expectancies similar to those in some of the world's least developed nations. Among other things, my work abroad had filled me with a basic curiosity for how the social and cultural aspects of a healthcare system should interact with its technical elements (e.g., clinical, economic). Furthermore, I had a clear sense of what the purpose of healthcare should be, and if enacted, what form street-level interactions with my patients and neighbors could take. In New York City the absence of interaction and investment between neighborhoods and the healthcare system is stark. This missing layer—which includes the fundamental role of community health workers abroad—could mobilize neighborhoods to undergo their own path to health improvement. But I also knew, from my experience across the MVP, that this was hard to do.

I had a lot to learn.

• • •

On July 1, 2011, I joined thousands of new interns across the country in my first year of an internal medicine residency at Mount Sinai Hospital in Manhattan, which included work in the Bronx Veterans Hospital and the city's Elmhurst Hospital in Queens. I began an unusual, half-time residency so I could simultaneously pursue scholarship and teaching as an assistant professor of international and public affairs at Columbia University. I made a case that the interactions between the healthcare system and its surrounding neighborhood was an underserved subject of analysis. I wanted to understand if there really was a missing layer, and if so, learn about it by trying to build it. Where to start?

In clinical training, you are constantly told to learn as much as you can from your patients. William Osler, one of four founding members of Johns Hopkins Hospital and considered a father of modern medicine, stated, "Listen to your patient, he is telling you the diagnosis."[7] This not only applies to the act of listening, but to the act of anchoring knowledge about the body, the healthcare system, and the world around the patient in one place in order to make an informed assessment. Unfortunately, the same care that is applied to the assessment of individual patients for their medical problems is rarely applied to how the healthcare system interacts with the places it serves.

The inspiration for this book is a patient who died under my care. He turned out to be a neighbor, as well, and I only really got to know him after he died. I refer to him as Ray.* His daughter unexpectedly invited me to his funeral, where I met his friends, family, and congregation. Like Ray, many of these people were living with chronic diseases and were unwell. I was puzzled by how a place so close to nine major regional hospitals, countless clinics, a world-famous public health department, and substantial social and economic investments could be so persistently unhealthy. How being part of a great American city, awash with wealth and opportunity, can merely be a noisy backdrop to the daily stress of life. In death, Ray began to show me a glimpse of healthcare in America that was visible only from the streets he walked. My work with CHWs across Africa had prepared me to see his world of the neighborhood and my world of the hospital as

---

* In order to maintain patient confidentiality, Ray is a composite of many patients, but all events and conversations are real.

interconnected, even if this connection was yet to be clearly defined. But it became obvious that if we did not build this connectivity and make it part of how we do healthcare in America, more of my neighbors would meet unnecessarily early deaths.

With real people in mind, the question shifts: how do *we* build this missing layer?

Acknowledgments

There are two sets of people for me to acknowledge: those who generously shaped my understanding of what this book should be as I wrote it, and those who made it possible for me to write it in the first place. Among the former are the people who appear in its pages, and the many more who patiently introduced new contexts and explained concepts: Ray and his daughter, in particular. The latter includes my mentors and family who moved mountains to give me the space and vantage point to undertake this effort. Together, they are inspiration, support, and encouragement embodied.

Every story has its origin, and this one was forged during an exhausting and exciting time as a clinical trainee at Mount Sinai Hospital, while I was also a young professor at Columbia University. This unusual arrangement was made possible by the shared vision of Paul Klotman and the late Mark Babyatsky at Mount Sinai, as well as Jeffrey Sachs and John Coatsworth of Columbia University. They supported the idea that my experience could be a laboratory for reflection, leading to the discovery of skills and insights unique to its context. At Mount Sinai Hospital, my colleagues and attendings inspired me to see the best in what healthcare could be. I have Jeffrey and Sonia Sachs to thank for nearly a decade of mentorship and for removing the barriers to making this unusual arrangement possible.

This book would not have been possible without the pivotal support of the Robert Wood Johnson Foundation, which introduced me to an extraordinary network of grantees, fellows, and practitioners across the country during their 40th anniversary celebration. In particular, Ruben Amarasingham, Ashley Atkinson, Scott Halpern, Naa Oyo Kwate, Raina Merchant, Rebecca Onie, Carmen Peralta, Doran Schrantz, Somava (Soma) Stout, and Robin Mockenhaupt. Alongside this group, I've consistently benefited from the wise counsel and writings of peers who helped me reflect upon the goals of this book. Liz Van Hoose and Anna Stapleton made my drafts more readable and helped me to untangle its structure.

On late night walks to my home in Harlem, with the lights of midtown Manhattan's skyscrapers in the receding distance, I often think about the journey my parents took from Nairobi, in search of opportunity and community. Their courage and determination are the bounce in my step, and my brother, Karan Dhadialla, a constant companion. Once I get home, however,

I'm immediately brought back to the present, where my elder son, Hukam Singh, bounds to the door, running ahead of his grandmother who holds our younger son, Vir Singh; they all remind me of just how blessed I am. At the end of the day, it is only fair that the last acknowledgment should go to my first reader, whose steadfast love and personal example always keep me striving to be a more thoughtful presence: Manmeet Kaur.

Chardi Kala!

Dying and Living in the Neighborhood

Introduction

In its current form, habits, and environment, American health care is incapable of providing the public with the quality health care it expects and deserves.
—Institute of Medicine, *Crossing the Quality Chasm*

If the American healthcare sector were a nation, it would be the sixth largest in the world by gross domestic product, sandwiched between France and Brazil.[1] It would have 27 million citizens, but no formal governance structure of its own.[2] Insurance company leaders, professional organization lobbyists, academic experts, hospital system administrators, shareholders in life science companies, and investors of private capital all play an outsize role in shaping its behavior. Although the healthcare sector is firmly embedded in the domestic affairs of American life, how are the more than 300 million Americans organized in this immense consolidation of economic activity? How is it possible for our collective and individual values and goals to enter this powerful mix? Is it even conceivable that a population of residents—the majority of whom lack deep technical knowledge of medicine, business insight into healthcare, or sufficient political clout to affect regulation—could change or improve how healthcare is structured? Who are the pioneers making this possible? Can their work be extended across the nation?

Designing a national healthcare system anywhere in the world is considered a "wicked problem," which Berkeley professors Horst W. J. Rittel and Melvin Webber defined in their famous paper on the topic: "Policy problems cannot be definitively described. Moreover, in a pluralistic society there is nothing like the undisputable public good; there is no objective definition of equity; policies that respond to social problems cannot be meaningfully correct or false; and it makes no sense to talk about 'optimal solutions' to social problems unless severe qualifications are imposed first."[3]

"Severe qualifications" may refer to strict limitations on the scope of a problem to be solved, the requirement that there only be one or a few sought-after outcomes, or a single guiding principle that focuses debate. I see the struggle over the definition of "value" in healthcare as the most consequential means of defining the scope, requirements, and aims of

1

healthcare reform. Today, "value" is most associated with financing and payment. While it is clear that healthcare financing needs an overhaul, such a shift alone is inadequate to address the deep disconnect between regional healthcare systems and the true drivers of health and prosperity in a given neighborhood.

When experts speak figuratively about making sure that healthcare sector participants have "skin in the game," it is easy to forget that patients always have skin in the game, literally. Put another way, a healthcare system that is imbalanced in favor of technocrats and captains of industry does not make a good neighbor to the more than 300 million Americans who are spread across 50 states, more than 3,000 counties, and 200,000 neighborhoods.* All Americans are stakeholders in the design and architecture of their healthcare system. Ignoring the places where we spend our lives in favor of a narrow focus on traditional, hospital- and clinic-based healthcare interactions is simply not a good sectorwide strategy.

And yet, it's the strategy that currently prevails. The creation, passage, and implementation of the 2010 Patient Protection and Affordable Care Act (ACA) was an exercise in expert design, agile legislative skill, and old-fashioned horse trading with incumbents. Its underlying goal was to slow the growth of healthcare spending while expanding healthcare insurance. The passage of the ACA was akin to watching an emergency room doctor at work. Whereas primary care physicians emphasize working with their patients to transform health guidelines into feasible everyday solutions, emergency room doctors need to rely on quick thinking and expert judgment to operate with minimal interference, lest they miss the lifesaving window of opportunity. In the primary care setting, trust and relationships are built over time; in the emergency room, trust is expended as loved ones watch helplessly. Although the ACA has coincided with what appears to be a temporary slowdown[4] in healthcare spending, it has increased healthcare insurance coverage. However, it is also among the most politically divisive legislation[5] since Medicare and Medicaid were enacted 50 years ago, in 1965. Most of us will never know what the ACA accomplished or forestalled, but we will remember that our communities were not included in the process. It is no surprise that support for healthcare reform remains deeply divided.[6]

---

* See below on my working definition of neighborhood, I use a census block as a proxy, simply to give a sense of scale in comparison to the 50 states and 3,144 counties.

But for all its controversy, the ACA does include elements that force the attention of healthcare system leaders outside the walls of the hospitals and clinics they oversee.

Over a hundred years ago, one of the founders of modern economics, Alfred Marshall, emphasized the advantage of seeing industry and neighborhood as linked and deeply interdependent:

> When an industry has thus chosen a locality for itself, it is likely to stay there long: so great are the advantages which people following the same skilled trade get from near neighborhood to one another. The mysteries of the trade become no mysteries; but are as it were in the air, and children learn many of them unconsciously. Good work is rightly appreciated, inventions and improvements in machinery, in processes and the general organization of the business have their merits promptly discussed: if one man starts a new idea, it is taken up by others and combined with suggestions of their own; and thus it becomes the source of further new ideas. And presently subsidiary trades grow up in the neighborhood, supplying it with implements and materials, organizing its traffic, and in many ways conducing to the economy of its material.[7]

If the *trade* is healthcare, and the *industry* is health improvement, Marshall's perspective is even more poignant in the context of recent work to clarify the term "neighborhood." Take the Urban Institute's 2014 description in *Strengthening Communities with Neighborhood Data*, for example:

> Typically referred to as neighborhoods within urban areas, they can also comprise villages or hamlets in rural areas. These areas are not simply geographic footprints but units of social organization that have meaning as places to live, work, and go about daily life. They have an identity in the minds of insiders and outsiders. Neighborhoods and villages are more than collections of individuals or locations for populations; they also include space, physical structures, social networks, formal and informal organizations, businesses, systems of exchange and governance, and so forth. These place-based communities are not islands, but are spatially located relative to other places. Moreover, they operate at various scales, from the immediate residential vicinity to wider areas of social, economic, and political relevance to daily life.[8]

We need to see neighborhoods as the primary infrastructure for improving health, rather than as landscapes that sit alongside—and outside—the healthcare systems that serve them. Americans' health, education, and prosperity are bound to where they live. In this broader context, hospitals and clinics play an important but limited role. With a rising epidemic of chronic medical conditions, both the social elements of health and the technical aspects of healthcare need to be better understood as parts of an integrated whole. When confronting a complex social issue like obesity, and the subsequent rise of a technical issue like diabetes management, it is clear that including the neighborhood in the context of designing a better healthcare system is more likely to address both. However, if the starting point for solutions lies within a healthcare system, potentially buried even more deeply within a laboratory, the neighborhood becomes an impossibly distanced abstraction. My own training as a physician-scientist heavily favored the laboratory-centric perspective.

One of my mentors was Jules Hirsch, a professor and physician-in-chief at Rockefeller University. In 1959 he began a pioneering series of experiments in metabolism and obesity that have personal and public implications even today. He persuaded eight people who had been obese since childhood to live in Rockefeller Hospital for eight months while they were studied intensely and fed about 600 calories of liquid a day, resulting in an average weight loss of 100 pounds.[9] None of us will be surprised to learn that most of the subjects rapidly regained the lost weight. It is precisely because of Hirsch's experiments that we know that our metabolism and will power are hardwired together and that dramatic weight loss is usually followed by equally dramatic weight gain. In the 1990s, another Rockefeller scientist, Jeffrey Friedman, began to unravel the tight linkage between genetics, behavior, and metabolism in obesity. Along with other researchers, he concluded that our genetic inheritance encoded our metabolic destiny in ways that would be extremely difficult to change. The best hope for an obese or diabetic patient would be a gastric bypass or maybe swapping out the bacteria in their gut. In this view, the mantra of diet and exercise is relatively futile.

Americans are intimately familiar with the flipside of these technical perspectives: obesity as a social issue, intimately linked to lifestyle and powerfully coupled to our local context. At some point between Hirsch's and Friedman's landmark experiments, Americans began to gain weight. Weight

Watchers became a cultural touchstone in the 1990s and airlines started charging very obese passengers for two seats. On the other hand, a fuller body was embraced as healthier and more natural in some communities— Peter Griffin in *The Family Guy* and Homer Simpson in *The Simpsons* both look pleasingly tubby. There is a lively debate about what is an optimal or unhealthy weight among healthcare experts, but the trend took on new, alarming significance when obesity was popularly noted to be rising in children at the turn of the twenty-first century.

Biomedical research could only provide a partial picture of what was going on. Economists conjectured that technologic change in the food industry had fueled a rise in calorie consumption, and food policy experts pointed to a dramatic rise in processed sugar. Apparently the food pyramid was a biased reflection of food industry lobbyists and misleading research. Our schools were stocked with sugary sodas and cheap, processed food, particularly in low-income neighborhoods. The association between obesity and the proximity of kids to parks, playgrounds, and healthy supermarkets painted a picture of our neighborhoods competing with our genetic inheritance for influence, compounded by a complex interplay of behavior and socioeconomics.[10] Public health practitioners had never lost sight of these complex societal factors, but only 3 percent of the nearly $3 trillion in healthcare spending goes their way, while community advocates fight an uphill battle to build a healthier neighborhood amidst tightening local budgets. In the clinical healthcare sector, increased sugar consumption was matched with insulin production and new classes of medication were rolled out to treat a rising epidemic of diabetes.

In 2002, the *New England Journal of Medicine* published a paper about a study to reduce the incidence of type 2 diabetes, the most common form of the disease.[11] Everyone in the study was at high risk for developing diabetes because they were obese, a condition shared by about one-third of all adult Americans (with more members of minority groups affected). One group got a diabetes medication called metformin along with the kind of diet and exercise advice you would find in a pamphlet, and another group was assigned a sixteen-lesson curriculum that was initially taught one-on-one so it could be tailored to the individual participants, followed by group sessions to reinforce behavior change. Unlike Hirsch's directives in the 1950s, the lifestyle changes advanced in the new study were modest—brisk walking for 2.5 hours a week and individually relevant dietary guidance that would achieve a 10-pound weight loss in a 150-pound person. After three years, both approaches reduced the incidence of diabetes, but the lifestyle change worked *twice* as well as the drug. People stuck to it. But in clinical health-care, the result was mostly greeted with, "That's nice, but who has the time to do the lifestyle intervention? It's hard enough to get patients to take their meds!" So, for the most part, clinicians have chosen to prescribe metformin, a solution that aligns with the structure of the American healthcare system no matter how inferior its logic and efficacy.

The growing dissonance between the structure and logic of healthcare and the needs of Americans to stay healthy inevitably leads to disillusion-ment by its professionals and distrust by the public. So why do we persist in this unsatisfactory state? The historian Charles Rosenberg captures the spirit of the "modern" physician's training:

> The vision looked inward toward the needs and priorities of the medical
> profession, inward toward the administrative needs of the individual hos-
> pital, inward toward a view of the body as a mechanism and away from that
> of the patient as social being and family member. It was a vision, moreover,
> so deeply felt as to preclude conscious planning, replacing it instead with
> a series of seemingly necessary actions. The decisions which shaped the
> modern hospital cannot be understood without an understanding of the
> peculiar world of medical ideas and values, what might be called the culture
> of medicine.[12]

The *culture of medicine* he refers to was from an article on the rise of the modern hospital from 1880 to 1914. It is no exaggeration, and even a source of professional pride, to say that this spirit has been conserved. However, as our burgeoning healthcare sector not only ignores the neighborhood, but constricts the investments that we can make to improve it, all of us, health-care professionals and the American public alike, have rightly perceived that the dissonance has grown too great, and at a huge cost.

During my internal medicine residency, I was steeped in the inward gaze of medicine. However, with the death of patients who crossed my path only in the advanced stages of a chronic illness, I also saw critical moments earlier in these patients' lives where the right support could have led to a very different outcome. But to meet people in these moments, when their minds are far away from the hospital or clinic, seemed like it would take an extraordinary reach. The irony is that as healthcare professionals, we pass by these moments regularly, as we walk to and from work and greet our friends and neighbors on the way.

By 2015, federal-level healthcare reform had definitively rolled out of Washington, DC, unfurling in substantively different ways across our 50 states and drawing attention of healthcare system leaders outward from the insular culture of medicine. In the streets outside the walls of our hospitals and clinics, there are schools, playgrounds, job training centers, and countless ways to be a part of a healthy community. How and if these neighborhood features fit into the structure and logic of healthcare transformed from a marginal notion into a pressing question. Whatever the fate of the ACA when its first implementers are no longer in office, there is no turning back from the inextricable link between life in the neighborhood and the health of our nation. The form and habits of healthcare need to be revised accordingly.

There will always be a role for clinic- and hospital-based healthcare, but it is time for it to shed some heft, and for healthcare to share in the work of building healthier neighborhoods. In this book, I set out to show that an expanded, yet more porous, view of a healthcare system is at hand, one that is guided by a strong public health system and anchored not in a hospital, but upon the infrastructure of a neighborhood in development. If this was simply a matter of coherent systems meeting one another, then the work ahead would be a function of visionary leadership, know-how, and execution. In reality, it's not so easy. Neighborhoods, and the healthcare and public health systems within them, present flashes of coherence as networks of organizational activity coalesce to solve specific problems, only to dissipate as a new need arises or the urgency to act systematically passes. The cost of managing this scatter is left to our neighbors across America, many of whom do not have the means or skills to assemble this activity into a coherent system that works for them.

The price of coherence is the active participation of Americans in the design of how healthcare systems interact with their neighborhoods. We resist the perception that our only role is as consumers and our only choices are those that govern healthcare's consumption. Today, however, we have little influence upon the architecture of healthcare itself. As a nation, we need to test, define, and augment the right combinations of organizations, social services, and small businesses that form a neighborhood-level health system, ones that can dissolve the walls of vertically integrated and narrowly networked healthcare systems that dominate the national landscape today. The engine of reform, new financial arrangements, management innovations, social technologies, and a new generation of inspirational pioneers are making this possible. However, our ability to maintain and improve our health, to redesign healthcare systems, and to discern the right architecture of healthcare's interaction with our neighborhoods is not a foregone conclusion. And at stake is nothing short of the health of our republic.

The methodology of this book is best understood as a problem- and solution-*seeking* effort, rather than a problem-*solving* one. One authoritative methodological source that influenced this book is *The Art of Systems Architecting*,[13] which draws upon the insights of engineers who found themselves trying to solve unprecedented problems that are social in nature. These challenges range from negotiating with politicians on the cost of a project—like a space shuttle—that neither side fully understands in advance, to scenarios where the "clients" of a complex system are scattered and diffuse—like Internet users. These engineers share "heuristics," practical approaches to problem solving that yield satisfactory and sufficient solutions that emerge as experts co-design systems with clients. Rather than viewing nontechnical participants as interfering, ignorant, or meddling, system architects embrace many perspectives. Herbert A. Simon, a Nobel Laureate in Economics and father of decision-making and organization theory, saw heuristics as a tool that all people use to build and design the complex organizations around them, whether they are aware of it or not.

Although heuristics have been studied at the clinician level, as in *How Doctors Think* by physician-writer Jerome Groopman, I have not encountered similarly thoughtful reflections on the heuristics that guide decision-making at the healthcare system level. Instead, we hear prescriptions, projections, and models, all in the domain of technical expertise, which force Americans to respond intuitively and emotionally, especially where they are missing information to respond more deliberately. In a narrative form, I search for a systems architecture that is both satisfactory and feasible in bridging the complex needs of healthcare systems and the neighborhood, starting with one person in one place to make the scope of the problem comprehensible. As I explore the context of a composite patient, I build heuristics to guide my search for people and places across the country that have constructive "views" on what a healthcare system ought to accomplish, even if they are not healthcare experts themselves. Lastly, I explore the tension between possible system designs that work best locally versus nationally and arrive at an architecture that enables search by local users across the country to find their own solutions. As I work through this process, my own biases and heuristics are exposed, with the hope that you, the reader, will see much to improve upon.

Part 1 of this book begins with the death of a patient I took care of in the hospital. "Ray" is a composite of four real people who all lived in the neighborhood of Harlem and shared similar life histories and clinical conditions. Demographically, he could have been a Robert or Ricardo, a Randall or Rahim. By creating a composite person I have complied with the letter and spirit of the confidentiality requirements in the Health Insurance Portability and Accountability Act (HIPAA). At the same time, this composite has allowed me to impart crucial personal details that form the bridge between a clinical setting and the neighborhood we shared. My curiosity as a physician trained to analyze and design systems led me to better understand how the neighborhood's healthcare and public health systems operated, or failed to do so, on the backdrop of decades of tumultuous economic development activity in the neighborhood.

In part 2, I report on the activity of nationally recognized pioneers who are acting on a local level across the country, building critical components of a neighborhood-based health system. In the process of my investigations, I encountered hundreds more people with similar visions of a porous, neighborhood-embedded healthcare system. I focus on just a few, who showed me how relationships—whether assigned by technology, forged by common struggle, or developed using formal or informal methods—form a powerful channel for simultaneously improving the health of neighborhoods while redesigning healthcare. Together these trailblazers are creating ways to connect and improve upon each other's insights in meaningful ways. What I find is not a set of prescriptions, but a growing national movement comprised of people who are redefining the boundaries and aim of American healthcare.

As individuals, we cannot create the conditions for a healthy and prosperous life independent of others. Neighborhoods are no different. In part 3, I explore how this movement to build a neighborhood-based health system is developing the structures it needs to be transformative: systematic ways

to learn from successes, new methods to connect and combine existing resources, and more responsive political and economic support to augment
local and regional democratic processes across the nation. In the Internet
age, it is perhaps no surprise that the metaphor of a network emerges as a
salient feature to emulate. The collaborative tenets applied to the creation
and modulation of Internet protocols have a vital place in the process of
architecting a new set of relationships between healthcare, public health,
and community development. Ultimately, I return to Harlem to see how we
might "plug in" to such a network. It is clear that the engine of a purposeful
redesign will have to be driven by my neighbors—and by my healthcare
colleagues and I as their neighbors—above all.

Healthcare is a complex system in transition, where the titanic movements
of its economic underpinnings have created unprecedented ambiguity
about what its future form will take. These are moments of systemic entrepreneurship, where the "right strategy" is ill defined and one person or
organization does not have the authority to define it. What emerges from
these historic moments is necessarily unprecedented, even if built upon
countless incremental, well-informed actions and activities. There is no
doubt in my mind that the structures we build will be rickety, and the logics we hew together will present many contradictions. But I feel confident
that in Harlem, my neighbors and my professional colleagues are not alone;
instead, we are among a nation of neighbors—both people and places—who
are emboldened to see an unprecedented future where Americans like Ray's
grandchildren are the healthiest generation we have yet to see.

Herein lies the basis of a purposeful exchange, one that I believe would
inspire even the most disillusioned healthcare practitioner, one that turns
anyone with the instinct for caregiving into an architect of reform: if we
take a little care to get to know those who share the same aims of a healthier
nation, the remedies we together devise will cure all sorts of illness.

I carry the memory of Ray as I move about our Harlem neighborhood
and across America. I am reminded of what Roger Cohen, a columnist, wrote
about his father when he died: "The living are the custodians of the souls of
the dead, those stealthy migrants. Love bequeaths this responsibility."[14] So
Harlem is where we begin and end, near the heart of *El Barrio*—"the neighborhood" within a nation of neighborhoods.

PART I

1

Out of Many, One

Insurance man, he did not pay–
His insurance lapsed the other day–
Yet they got a satin box
For his head to lay
—Langston Hughes, "Night Funeral in Harlem"

THE FUNERAL

It is unusual for a clinical trainee to attend the funeral of a patient who has died in the hospital, despite the intense interaction that can occur with patients and their families in the critical care setting. We pronounce their physical death but are rarely privy to the impact of their passing in their own community. Their body is cremated or buried, their clinical records are transcribed into an official death record, but the personal consequence of death and its social expression are considered beyond the scope of clinical interest. In the blur of medical school, it almost feels like the entire world comes to the hospital door—babies and mothers, adults, the elderly. It is easy to confuse the emotion and intensity of life in the hospital with the world around it.

Despite the fact that my patient Ray was also my neighbor, his world turned out to be as foreign to me, his doctor, as the language of my hospital world was to his daughter. Our neighborhood, referred to as *El Barrio* ("the neighborhood"), is part of a cluster of historic Harlem neighborhoods. If you were flying into one of the two nearby New York City airports, Ray's Harlem apartment building would be difficult to identify among the grid of blocks and superblocks that blend into the rest of the city. Unless you grew up in the area, you wouldn't necessarily be able to distinguish the western border of East Harlem from Central Harlem, or the southern border of East Harlem from the Upper East Side. Only a history whiz would know that the superblocks are the most visible expression of the vast public works projects built over half a century ago. A dwindling number of old-timers recall life before the projects, when your street was your universe and waves of immigrants found their economic footing in America and then promptly dispersed to the suburbs.

Today, word on the street is that upper Manhattan is a good place to buy property. "Infilling" is the new buzzword for repurposing urban space and countering suburban sprawl. In practice, it has meant that my family had an opportunity to move into a nice apartment that is expensive for the neighborhood but cheap for Manhattan. Real estate prices are rising rapidly and multi-million-dollar brownstones are sold for cash within days of being listed, often purchased by foreign investors and anonymous financial entities. The crumbling project buildings, grandly named after famous Americans—Washington, Jefferson, Taft, Wilson, Wagner—are visible reminders that a rising tide of prosperity doesn't automatically lift all boats. I had been so busy with clinical training that I had barely met the people on my apartment floor, much less people in my new neighborhood.

Ray's daughter reached out to me after his death. The relationship we had forged during his treatment inspired her to invite me to his funeral. As I listened to Ray's eulogy along with his family members and friends, I could feel the thick social structure of the community. The wooden pews held Ray's fellow veterans in uniform and his grandchildren all dressed in dark blue; there were clusters of generations, leaning on canes or hunched over smartphones. In the hospital—where Ray was attended to by white coat–clad doctors, blue-smocked patient care assistants, and nurses in color-coded uniforms that designated their area—I could probably tell you what was going on just by noting the clinicians assembled around a patient. Here in Ray's church, I realized I did not know my neighbors well enough to do the same. Instead, I sat quietly in the last row of pews as the pastor made a brief reference to Ray's health, explaining, "He knew that going to the hospital meant trouble, and so he waited and waited until it was absolutely necessary." I slowly realized that in Ray's view, a doctor's diagnosis signaled the *creation* of a problem.

But from my perspective as a doctor, his delay in getting medical care for a chronic condition was the true source of that trouble. According to the records I had available, his most common form of transportation to the hospital was an ambulance. His last lab values were years old, and the records we had faxed to us indicated that he had had many different primary care doctors. When we conducted a new set of tests to establish how far Ray's chronic medical conditions had progressed, it was clear that he had a systemwide challenge in his body. As I sat in pews where Ray had sat while he was alive, I realized we were looking at the same challenge through completely different perspectives. How could this difference have been bridged?

The progression of chronic conditions is gradual; it is difficult for most people to distinguish clinical worsening from a new normal. If most of the people around you have swollen legs or seem to be taking more pills with the passing years, it's easier to view these symptoms as the expected accompaniments to aging, rather than as evidence of ill health.

I encountered Ray only after this gradual progression had become acute. As the heat in Harlem reached its apex in the summer of 2011, a small clot began to form in the vein of Ray's right thigh. Like a fan stoking embers, his heart fluttered irregularly, creating the turbulent conditions for the clot to grow. Just a few days before he came under my care, paramedics had taken him to the emergency room of Harlem Hospital after his blood sugar had dropped dangerously low. He recovered after getting some sugar and was discharged with a note instructing him to reduce his insulin dose. After leaving that hospital, he had spent his time sitting on the couch at home, listlessly staring past daytime television. His daughter spoke to him over the phone but didn't succeed in getting him to the senior center for company. She was exhausted from the stress and anxiety of caring for him and promised herself she would visit soon. Meanwhile, fluid pooled in Ray's lower legs as his heart weakly pumped, rendered less effective by its irregular rhythm. All the while, the clot in his right thigh vein migrated hurriedly in the direction of his heart, threatening to whoosh into his lungs and tip his heart into failure.

Ray's daughter checked in on him the next day and knew something was wrong: he ignored news about his favorite granddaughter. After cleaning up empty Chinese food boxes, she left to get him some more food. As she returned, paramedics were entering the building. She knew they were coming for him. As they were transferring him to a stretcher, she saw his insulin pen resting on a nearby shelf. He had finally gotten around to using the insulin pen, adjusting its dial by himself for the first time in years. He accidentally turned it the wrong way. A little while after, he lost consciousness and fell to the floor. Ray's apartment door was open, as it had been every day for many years, and a neighbor heard a thud as he banged his right thigh on the way down.

At Mount Sinai's emergency room, we tried to piece together his clinical state: Ray had uncontrolled diabetes, which is the leading cause of kidney failure. High blood pressure is both a cause and consequence of this process. As a heart beats under higher pressures, it can enlarge and stiffen. If the heart weakens substantially, fluid backs up into places like the legs, lungs, and liver. All bets are off when its ability to keep a regular beat goes haywire. Smoking makes *everything* worse as a legacy of toxins leaves an indelible mark. Even though Ray had quit smoking more than a decade before, his body showed the evidence. Family genetics encode another layer of explanation that clinicians are only beginning to understand. Most of Ray's medical conditions were interrelated in ways that clinician-scientists have teased out through decades of research, built upon the powerful precept that everything in the mind and body is connected at some level, even if we do not yet know how. For all we could hypothesize, test, manage, and treat, his clinical course had been set in motion decades before he entered our care.

Ten days later, he was dead.

As I stood in the church lobby, Ray's family members stopped to speak with me. They were curious about my presence and made me feel welcome. They talked to me about Ray as if I had known him intimately. He had served in Vietnam, but ever since returning to civilian life he had struggled to make a living. He held temporary jobs, punctuated by increasingly long periods of unemployment. At some point he just stopped looking for work because people questioned why he had not held a job. His wife, a secretary, was deeply involved in church life, but she found it challenging to keep him engaged. He never got over the active participation of black churches against the Vietnam War, despite meeting his wife at a church event. One of his teenage granddaughters told me that he was a wonderful storyteller when he felt up to it, although he had rarely spoken in recent years. His son said that he had difficulty reading, which no one had noticed until Ray started having trouble paying bills after his wife died. Some assumed he was illiterate, but could it have been his declining eyesight? They asked me to speculate. (I did not know.)

The rent-controlled apartment that he called home for 40 years is part of a superblock in East Harlem, which hosts one of the highest densities of urban housing projects in America. After Ray came back from the war, he was mugged frequently and became wary of leaving his home. Even though security in the neighborhood has improved dramatically over the past 20 years, police presence in an area with a high concentration of methadone clinics did little to encourage him to step outside. His wife had been his lifeline to the world beyond the apartment. After she died, he barely ventured out of his building. I imagined him sitting in his apartment waiting for time to pass as high-end condos sprang up around him and different wars filled the evening news. I had trained for a decade, preparing to be his doctor— preparing to meet him only in sickness, not in health.

Before I left the funeral, I spoke to the pastor about his perspective on the health of his congregation. He gently explained how part of his job is to support his congregation when he senses trouble. He is worried about obesity in kids and how to counsel middle-aged couples when a spouse needs to start dialysis. He explained that his congregation does not always make distinctions between spiritual support and clinical decision-making, and he has had to manage it all. He had caught wind of a new Department of Health and Mental Hygiene program in Brooklyn that helped pastors like him, but could not find any information online.[1] In the lead of a vibrant congregation and amidst a dense cluster of public health programs, social services, and hospitals, Ray's pastor felt alone.

Etched into the design of our healthcare system is the basic assumption that when people like Ray get sick enough, they will come our way. Once they are with us, protocols will be followed, evidence applied, actions coded and billed, and, for the most part, textbook healthcare delivered. When I think back to our clinical interaction, Ray and I played our roles flawlessly. Despite occasionally getting fed up or irritated by the instructions his doctors gave him, he felt obligated to follow them, and to show up when instructed. As I reflected upon Ray's death in my hospital and his funeral in our neighborhood, a line that the physician Paul Farmer wrote resonated deeply with me: "It is our collective practice that is malpractice."[2]

I paid my respects to the well-dressed man in the coffin. I recognized him from his exposed ankles, located between short tan stocks and neatly pressed beige dress pants, where his skin was darkened and wrinkled from years of blood pooling in his legs. I had seen his exposed chest prior to his being transferred to the intensive care unit (ICU); now I saw a cream-colored silk tie rest upon a dark brown vest, with an unwound pocket watch frozen at ten past two. I realized I did not really know anything about him, or his life. In the hospital, this fact just did not seem important. In front of him now, it felt disrespectful. If the healthcare system and neighborhood both care about his well-being, why are they so evidently disconnected?

A GROWING SENSE OF DISTANCE

If we glance at the developments of the past century that have contributed to our current healthcare architecture, there are clues as to where and when its design sharply diverged from its broader social context. Despite the current separation of healthcare and neighborhood, the two were not always necessarily seen as distinct. S. S. Goldwater, superintendent of Mount Sinai Hospital and widely considered the nation's first professional medical administrator, established a Social Service Department, which was lauded in the hospital's 1908 annual report. "It is now recognized that the condition of a patient's family while he is in our wards, as well as his needs immediately after his discharge from the hospital, constitute so vital a part of his ability to recover, and to retain his health, that the work of this department has come to be recognized as a legitimate part of the functions of the institution."[3]

However, this emphasis was overshadowed by the formalization of scientific approaches to medical care. Goldwater's vision would recede to the margins of hospital administration for more than a century. Just a couple of years after that 1908 annual report, the hospital's Social Service Department fell out of vogue, supplanted by the zeitgeist surrounding the influential Flexner report (1910), which had been commissioned by the Carnegie Foundation and authored by education reformer Abraham Flexner. He was an admirer of the German approach to scientific medical education, which was shaped by historic figures like Rudolph Virchow, who had made seminal discoveries in the biological basis of disease. Without taking into account Germany's sociopolitical context, where figures like Virchow were intensely active, the Flexner report emphasized the role of scientific thought, hospital-based training, and licensing requirements. Part of Flexner's goal was to stamp out what he considered to be a proliferation of unconscionably low-quality approaches to medical training, by appointing gatekeeper institutions. Abraham Flexner's brother, Simon, was the first director of the Rockefeller Institute for Medical Research (later renamed Rockefeller University), and channeled the Rockefeller family's fortune in a manner complementary to Carnegie's. The marriage of financial muscle, growing political influence, and mission-driven research ignited an era of biomedical innovation, reinvestment, and industrialization.

The steady stream of practical biomedical discoveries were not framed in opposition to the physician's social mission; in fact, the Flexner report made explicit reference to a physician as a "social instrument." Many early scientific discoveries in hygiene, sanitation, and public health could be easily coded as "social innovations," but the context for these pursuits was not at all social. It was the hospital, where patients could be carefully studied in an isolated setting. Venerable medical institutions like Johns Hopkins and the Columbia College of Physicians and Surgeons exemplify the biomedical model that still defines healthcare today: factories of medical innovation relatively isolated from the struggling neighborhoods surrounding them.

In the decades following Flexner's report, Mount Sinai Hospital came to exemplify the Germanic model as a wave of leading Jewish physicians and scientists joined the staff after fleeing Germany's rising anti-Semitism. The 1930 Ransdell Act established the federally funded National Institute of Health, which would expand to encompass a smattering of institutes that still reflect the human body as a project to be deconstructed into its component parts and biological disorders: eye, heart, cancer, arthritis and musculoskeletal skin diseases, neurological disorders and stroke, and so on. The model has been extraordinarily successful, despite requiring regular efforts to reform its sprawling structure and patchy performance. Antibiotics, anesthetics, and new diagnostic capabilities heralded a march of discovery and cure, triumphing over acute conditions that had previously killed patients overnight. The biomedical model of laboratory-driven research and discovery, followed by bedside treatment, came to be seen as the primary social mission of the hospital physician.

In the 1940s, Ray had emigrated north with his parents and extended family, where they found jobs in factories and hospitals. By 1959, when Ray was a teenager, Harlem's Jewish population had dwindled, along with that of other ethnic groups that had prospered in the early twentieth century. Although Mount Sinai Hospital continued to serve the neighborhood, its doctors and administrators increasingly lived elsewhere. Hospital workers with nonclinical roles were mostly African Americans and Puerto Ricans who lived nearby. That year, they began organizing for better pay and working conditions under a small union called the Local 1199. They found strong support among civil rights, human rights, and political leaders such as Martin Luther King Jr., Eleanor Roosevelt, and Adam Clayton Powell Jr., respectively. They felt it was their moral imperative to stage a strike to highlight the need for better conditions.

Yet the hospital also claimed righteousness in opposing a strike. At the time of the strike, the director of Mount Sinai Hospital, Martin Steinberg, stated, "A hospital is not an economic, industrial unit . . . it is a social unit . . . Human life should not be a pawn in jousting for economic gain or power."[4] He was speaking for his patients, who stood apart, in his mind, from the health and prosperity of the neighborhood workers who participated in their care. The "social unit" that he referred to included both clinical services and biomedical research, such as the nation's second blood bank and its first-ever published description of Crohn's disease. From Steinberg's perspective, the social unit of the hospital had the potential to transcend the particularities of a place like Harlem in the greater service of humanity. Capitulating to the demands of hospital workers would diminish its potential, and the strike was seen as an ethical affront to the hospital's social mission. Although I can empathize with Steinberg's analysis, he overlooked the fact that patients and the hospital's workers, nearly all of them neighbors, were inextricably linked.

Both sides claim that year's 46-day strike as a victory. The 1199's successfully organized effort powered the growth of today's 360,000-strong Service Employees International Union (SEIU), while the highly coordinated and well-prepared response of the hospitals in New York strengthened the Greater New York Hospital Association. Patient care was minimally disrupted and workers earned the right to organize. And yet, the distance between the neighborhood and the hospital grew.

BEYOND THE WALLS

Throughout the second half of the twentieth century, pioneering healthcare professionals made notable efforts to bridge the widening gap between clinical settings and the neighborhood. The same year Martin Luther King Jr. denounced the Vietnam War in a historic address at Harlem's Riverside

Church, a young doctor named Harold P. Freeman finished his training in surgical oncology at Memorial Sloan Kettering Cancer Center. Freeman came from an accomplished African American family that included his cousin Robert Weaver, who was the first secretary of the Department of Housing and Urban Development (HUD) and first African American member of the president's cabinet. Freeman could have gone anywhere in the country, but he headed a few miles uptown to Harlem Hospital Center. It was 1967, and Ray was deployed in South Vietnam with the US Army. As Martin Luther King Jr. drew parallels between the war abroad and poverty at home, Freeman was trying to understand how to translate the cutting-edge training he had received to the patients he was encountering in Harlem.

The techniques Freeman had learned were predicated upon early detection and treatment, which were largely irrelevant for the advanced cases of cancer he regularly encountered: "Technology was not the fundamental answer for the community I was dealing with; what I really needed to know was, why do people come in too late for treatment?"[5] Instead of simply offering the best he could for patients who showed up to the hospital, he immersed himself in the community and embarked on historic explorations of the links between poverty and cancer.[6] Through a series of landmark studies that drew upon the participation of community members across Harlem, he showed that social, economic, and cultural barriers led to delays in diagnosis and treatment of breast cancer, which substantially increased mortality.

While Dr. Freeman was developing his ideas in the 1970s, Ray had returned from Vietnam to a neighborhood in deep distress. In a sermon cited by a 1978 *New York Times* article, Rev. Robert Chapman referenced a famous poem by Langston Hughes, Harlem's poet laureate, when he lamented, "Harlem is that broken-winged bird. Its dreams are dead, its people are despairing and worse off than they ever were, and all the high hopes of the 1960s are gone."[7] The reverend could have been speaking about much of the country, as the national "misery index" (unemployment + inflation) reached an all-time high.

As the neighborhood's economy imploded, jobs were scarce and unemployment soared. For Harold Freeman, Harlem's deteriorating condition made it easier to see that healthcare was never just about discovering medicines or devising ingenious surgeries: "We generally talk of the war against cancer like it's a research war [however, it] needs to be fought in the neighborhoods where people live and die."[8] Although he studied cancer, he knew that people in the neighborhood were dying too young across the board. In 1990, he published a landmark article in the *New England Journal of Medicine* with his colleague Colin McCord. "Excess Mortality in Harlem" concluded "that Harlem and probably other inner-city areas with largely black populations have extremely high mortality rates that justify special consideration analogous to that given to natural disaster areas."[9]

In my view, Harold Freeman is the embodiment of the promise health-care could hold—someone who entered into a poorly understood domain because his purpose required it. Instead of waiting in his operating room to practice the sort of heroism attributed to uncommon skill and medical technology, he moved beyond the walls of the hospital. He made a feared and stigmatized illness comprehensible to the people who experience it. He recognized the power of cultural knowledge and local experience in ways he had never learned in medical school. He understood that healthcare was not an endpoint, and therefore was able to both improve upon it and transcend its limitations.

After decades of work to understand the problem, Freeman established the nation's first "Patient Navigator" program in 1990. The initial focus was upon reducing the critical time period between noting troubling symptoms and commencing appropriate treatment.[10] The key to his program was training people from the neighborhood to make sure that someone who had symptoms suspicious of breast cancer got through a gauntlet of tests and evaluations. At the time, navigators did not have the data, communication technologies, or evidence to guide their work. It may seem intuitive that if someone is concerned about their health, they would be proactive about seeking care. But to patients who may have felt fine, the difference between two and four weeks between appointments, for instance, didn't seem to matter. In aggressive cancers, however, time is of the essence, and the risk of spread to other parts of the body grows by the day. The patient navigator approach is a "patient-centric delivery model [that] serves to virtually integrate the fragmented healthcare system for the individual patient."[11] In other words, it took an experienced guide to make sure that patients did not get lost in a labyrinth of hospitals and clinics. It likely had some impact: in 1964, 49 percent of women in the community with breast cancer presented in late stages, compared to 21 percent between 1995 and 2000.[12]

However, in Harlem and across the nation, innovative neighborhood-based programs like this have had limited historical support to spread or scale. Without the full strength of investment and interest that traditional biomedical research and hospital-based clinical systems have enjoyed, efforts like this have not gone through a rapid progression of rigorously identifying their active ingredients, generalizing them beyond a handful of contexts, building systems and technologies to support efficient implementation and geographic spread, and, finally, identifying their limitations as the basis of further development. Even today, they lag behind the sophisticated community health worker management systems I saw and helped to build across sub-Saharan Africa, where the concept of community-based accompaniment is integral, not ancillary, to how healthcare systems function.

After 40 years of sustained effort, Dr. Freeman's work formed the basis of the Patient Navigator Outreach and Chronic Disease Prevention Act (2005), which was signed into law by President George W. Bush. The law was a gesture of recognition for Freeman's work, which led to a scattering of modestly funded pilot programs. Unfortunately, these were implemented without a path to sustainability. Health in Harlem remained poor.

The same year the Navigator Act was passed, a group of residents, activists, and Mount Sinai academics came together to form Help Educate to Eliminate Diabetes (Project HEED). In a study led by Project HEED, more than 70 percent of East Harlem residents had diabetes or prediabetes,[13] and nearly the same percentage were overweight or obese.[14] In the words of a pastor who was part of the group, "I feel like the people in our community are walking toward a cliff, and we need to join together, put our arms around them and pull them back."[15] The Project HEED team identified multiple factors that make it challenging for their neighbors with diabetes to eat in a healthy manner, including low consumption of healthy foods, clinicians who were rarely able to explain how they should eat, impatience for results (healthy eating does not lead to immediate changes in how a person feels), and chronic stress that worsened unhealthy eating.[16]

As the Project HEED team attempted to address these factors in a participatory manner, a small but significant national movement was afoot to explicitly bridge healthcare with neighborhood support services. For example, the national nonprofit Health Leads began placing volunteers who connect patients to support services in the pediatric clinic waiting room of Harlem Hospital pediatric clinics in 1999. It took another ten years to add one more desk to the obstetrics clinic. Now, when an overweight or diabetic patient enters the clinic, the electronic health record automatically prints a prescription for Health Leads. From there, volunteers work with patients to understand their social circumstances and actively connect them with neighborhood resources that they probably never knew existed. As Health Leads founder Rebecca Onie says, "In the private sector, when you squeeze that kind of additional value out of a fixed-cost investment, it's called a billion-dollar company. In my world, it's called reduced obesity and diabetes. It's called healthcare, a system where doctors can prescribe solutions to improve health, not just manage disease."[17]

When the 2010 Affordable Care Act (ACA) announced financial penalties for high rates of frequent readmission to the hospital, healthcare facilities like Mount Sinai stood to lose millions of dollars as nearly a third of the patients it treated for conditions like heart failure bounced back within days. Fortunately, neighborhood-centric healthcare had not been completely discarded; it was simply taking place in the margins outside biomedical research and hospital-based investments. In 2012, Mount Sinai announced that the Institute for Family Health, a network of 27 community health centers (CHC) with a significant Harlem presence, would form the basis of a new Department of Family Medicine and Community Health. Back in the 1960s, simultaneous to Harold Freeman's work in Harlem, physician H. Jack Geiger and colleagues Count Gibson and John W. Hatch founded the CHC movement by establishing the Delta Health Center, 1,200 miles away in Mound Bayou, Mississippi. The concept was simple—create health centers that are calibrated to the needs of the community. The idea was that CHCs would address the primary causes of poor health, even if they were socially rooted. When asked why Geiger was writing prescriptions for food, he famously responded, "Last time I checked my textbooks the specific therapy for malnutrition was, in fact, food."[18] Their work inspired a national network of nearly 10,000 CHCs across America. After nearly a century hiatus, hospitals across the country, like Mount Sinai under Goldwater's influence, were confronting the insidious gap with their neighborhoods: they found promising pieces of an incomplete puzzle.

Yet none of these repeated, isolated attempts to bridge the divide between healthcare and the neighborhood had any hope of impacting Ray in time. While Freeman's concept was evolving, my patient began developing symptoms of conditions that would eventually lead him to frequent, disconnected hospital encounters starting in the 1990s. Unlike the women who were at the center of Freeman's efforts to bridge the gap between symptoms and treatment of breast cancer, or the Project HEED community members in East Harlem, or the pediatric and obstetrics patients who benefited from Health Leads volunteers, Ray was left to find his own way.

DOUBLE-BLIND ENCOUNTERS

In the summer of 2011, I was in the first month of my internal medicine residency, frantically trying to keep up with the fast pace of Mount Sinai Hospital. I first met Ray in our crowded Emergency Department (ED) where transport beds were double-parked in the hallways. Most of the patients on these beds wore standard-issue hospital gowns over their street clothes, filling the room with hues of dull blue, accented by muted diagonal stripes printed on distressed cotton. Ray's eyes were glazed and his lips dry. Just a few days had passed since he had been released from a neighboring hospital. He seemed to slur his speech when he spoke, but it was hard to tell. The ED doctors noted the same thing and had sent him for a CT scan of his head before our internal medicine team had even seen him. There was no evidence that he had suffered a stroke. I diligently crossed "CVA" (shorthand for stroke) off the list of dangerous conditions we were told never to miss.

Ray's daughter returned to his side after finishing paperwork. He stared absently ahead. I addressed my questions to her as I gathered his history in the structured way that all doctors are taught. Through a series of directed questions, I filtered what she told me onto a piece of paper folded in half three times, creating a total of 16 boxes, each representing one patient. On it, I used a litany of abbreviations to record history and lab values and to build a to-do checklist. This information would quickly make its way into an electronic template that drives treatment decisions, consultation by specialists, and billing by the hospital.

Medical Record Number / Name: # / Ray

Chief Complaint: Syncope

History of Present Illness: ## yo M obese, IDDM, HTN, CKD,
    CHF (LVEF 45%), PAF ?AC . . .

Past Medical History: per HPI

Past Surgical History: distant removal of shrapnel s/p right side
    chest tube, right ORIF (90's)

Social History: widower, daughter is HCP, former smoker
    (30 pack year), no IVDU, ?alcohol
Allergies: NKDA
Medications: . . .

As I got up to speed, his daughter told me that his southern drawl became more pronounced when he was sick or tired. He was originally from
North Carolina, but this piece of information didn't make the cut for formal
documentation purposes. Nor did the promise she asked me to make: "Last
year Mama came into the hospital just like [he] does now, and the next
thing you know, she was in the intensive care unit and dying. We prayed for
a miracle, but you weren't able to save her—I don't think you even figured
out how she died. Promise this isn't that."

I had to take a step back. I did not know what was wrong with Ray.

His daughter spoke to me as if I were answering for every clinician who
ever knew Ray and every interaction with the healthcare system he had had.
As if all the information that hundreds of clinicians and care workers had
diligently asked of him and his family over the past decades were somehow
in my possession. In truth, I knew next to nothing about him, and what I
could know was scant. What I had was the strongly held belief by my profession that his presence in front of me was enough to go on, and that my laying
of hands upon him and a scatter of clinical diagnostics would establish what
was normal or abnormal about him. We are taught to look at patients with
fresh eyes, through the narrow aperture of their current clinical context. I
began to build a set of possibilities of what was wrong with him, from the
most to least likely, as well as the most to least dangerous, and began to
test him against these frameworks. Based upon the information I gathered
about him at our first meeting, I had to develop a hypothesis about what
his body would do next, so we could stop, manage, extract it, or in some way
intervene.

People enter healthcare systems without a clear understanding of what
will happen to them. The most powerful driver of activity in the clinical
world is that time may be of the essence. As a result, the overwhelmed and
busy new trainee operates under the point of view that if decline is not
imminent, patients and their family should be calm and understanding as
a structured diagnostic process unfolds. Clinicians condense the collective
intuition of their specific field, comprised of accessible evidence, inherited

wisdom, and personal experience, and bring it to bear upon the person in front of them. With so much to integrate upon meeting a person like Ray, it is easy to confuse evidence-based methods with ritual activity, to confuse the work of caregiving with unthinkingly following procedure. A web of clinical staff ranging from medical technicians to nurse managers watch over hundreds of parallel processes and overlapping workflows that form invisible barriers separating the lay from the expert.

Together, EDs and clinics do their best to discern which patients would benefit from hospitalization—with all its costs and collateral risks—and who within the hospital should preside over their care. In the process, loved ones are introduced to a technical language that predominates in a system where healthcare professionals are native and patients are foreign. As Susan Sontag, a writer who became a patient at Memorial Sloan Kettering Cancer Center when I was a medical student, wrote, "illness is the night side of life, a more onerous citizenship."[19] In these terms, a modern-day healthcare professional thrives in the night side of life, an inverted world where we gather constellations of data to navigate patients to safe harbor *within* the healthcare system. In contrast, to extend Sontag's metaphor, a *less* onerous citizenship is a path of health, self-illuminated by the aims and obligations of life in our neighborhoods, where a heavy fog of complexity stymies healthcare professionals.

In his 1992 *New York Times* review of I. M. Pei's newly unveiled Guggenheim Pavilion on Mount Sinai Hospital's campus, the critic Herbert Muschamp speaks in admiring terms about how the hospital melds with its surroundings: "The interplay between interior and exterior space creates an apt metaphor for the hospital as a place where people withdraw and prepare to rejoin the life of the city."[20] Indeed, in a hospital, a person's identity in the cultural or civic life of their neighborhood or nation—beloved grandfather or local leader—is quickly overshadowed by his role as a patient. If people are fortunate enough to leave the hospital, their role as a patient is quickly diminished by their return to the neighborhood, with the responsibilities and relationships therein. This binary also encodes the limited view of a hospital's role in a neighborhood—as a place of refuge, research, and repair, but an otherwise passive force in the health of its neighbors. As our neighbors become our patients, they are determined to glean enough about our arcane systems to convey their goals and aspirations in our terms. And so they guess, demand, and hope, inevitably falling short of their intent.

So when Ray's daughter asked me to promise that her father's stay at the hospital would not end in an unexplained death, as her mother's had— a lot of healthcare that yielded little enlightenment or comfort—I did not know what to say. Maybe he had a minor infection that was clouding his thinking, or maybe he was dying. There was no use speculating when there was so much we did not know. My mind was already ricocheting between disparate pieces of data that needed to be stitched together into a clinical workflow.

In the four years following Ray's death, my training in internal medicine was an extended drill in separating the knowable from what we clinicians consider unknowable or not worth knowing. At first, the extraordinary range of ways that the same category of acute sickness, syndrome, or condition could manifest in different patients was dizzying. As I progressed, however, I learned to pay closer attention to things like the fullness in patients' neck veins, the convexity of their temples, the curvature of their nails, the subtle sound of harsh rubbing as their heart beat, along with laboratory data and radiologic imaging. I constantly referenced a rapidly evolving set of guidelines while conferring with senior doctors as I developed my own understanding of what I could do when patients tip into "florid" illness or experience "indolent" decline. Although there are many healthcare professionals on a patient care team—multiple levels of nurses, physician assistants, diagnostic technicians, and so on—I was so absorbed with my own work that I barely registered their integral role in caring for our shared patient.

Instead, my more steady companions were the symptoms that the patient manifested and the constant stream of data that informed decision-making on daily rounds that could last hours. A brief summary of our plan would be conveyed to the patient at some point in the day, when there was time. On average, a first-year clinical resident spends about 8 minutes per a roughly 14-hour day with each of his 10 to 20 patients.[21] I began to understand what the "internal" part of "internal medicine" conveyed; akin to what influential philosopher Michel Foucault called the "medical gaze": "Facilitated by the medical technologies that frame and focus the physicians' optical grasp of the patient, the medical gaze abstracts the suffering person from her sociological context and reframes her as a 'case' or a 'condition.'"[22]

By the middle of my residency, the inner workings of different hospitals were more familiar to me than the common arrangement of products in bodegas across my neighborhood. Compared with the time when I met Ray, when I was disoriented by the newness of the environment and intimidated by hundreds of healthcare professionals intensely engaged in their tasks, the workflows of different hospitals took on a unified feel. Along the way, I learned to treat most nonclinical information as noise. If a piece of data did not directly contribute to the diagnosis and management of my patient, I did my best to ignore it so I would not miss something that endangered the patient. The outside world rarely intruded upon my focus on mastering clinical workflows: I only learned about the impending Hurricane Sandy that crushed New York City and the Tri-State area in the fall of 2012 through an email from the hospital about readiness activities. Otherwise I might not have noticed.

In exchange for blinders to the outside world, I began to learn the trade of healthcare delivery: the modern clinician translates a patient's symptoms into the language of their subspecialty, which then can be further translated into a standard syntax of healthcare codes and protocols. Possessing a highly technical language is both reassuring and dangerous. Every statement is imbued with a sense of purpose, with the assumption that omissions are purposeful. These statements are then amplified, copied, evolved, and even accidentally mutated as the responsibility for caregiving is distributed across an increasingly complex set of healthcare system actors. As a result, a patient or caregiver has no choice but to trust in the system, and its ability to produce accurate, pertinent information. But Ray's experience makes clear that such trust is not always deserved.

Ray's hospitalization in the 1990s, for dehydration and very high blood sugar levels, was also when he was first diagnosed with diabetes. The way his family tells it, he was discharged from the hospital without being told about his new diagnosis. And so less than two weeks later, he was hospitalized again for the same reasons. During his second hospitalization, he insisted that someone explain what it meant to be diabetic. After he left the hospital the second time, he wanted to stay out. But he soon found out that the medications he was getting were not putting him on the road to a cure. He had found the short lectures in the doctor's office about lifestyle change irritating, and at home, he took medications only when he noticed symptoms. His daughter recalled that every time he reluctantly went to the doctor, they diagnosed him with a new disease—first his sugar, then his blood pressure, next his kidney, and also his heart. Eventually, he was told he was depressed on top of everything else, and he vowed never to go back. Who could blame him?

It is not hard to imagine that as the list of Ray's interrelated conditions began to grow, he bounced from specialist to specialist, all of whom did their part without fully integrating what had come before or anticipating what he should do next. Today, healthcare system leadership would likely prefer their institutions be viewed as an interlocking matrix of highly trained individuals, disease-focused programs, and systemwide initiatives. In this view, symptoms and diagnostic data are coded into medical language that facilitates measurement and feedback to guide management and treatment. In contrast to this orderly view, Americans justifiably regard the hospital like a busy Old World bazaar, where guilds of specialists rent space, and the hospital serves as a landlord that makes sure there are heads in beds.

Ray's daughter felt blind, unable to do her part to navigate her father to safe harbor, which she regarded as bringing him home, not having him die in the hospital. So it is only fair that I was asked to make a promise, to break through the wall of the professional-client dynamic to speak person to person. It would not have been hard for me to promise Ray's daughter that her father's illness was different from her mother's, even without knowing anything about her. How people die, exactly, is like a fingerprint—there are common patterns, but we rarely know, precisely, what physical circumstances cause a particular death. Potential nonphysical contributors like socioeconomic status, pattern of behaviors, or the living environment are considered out of scope if they reside beyond the clinical sphere of influence.

These distinctions would have made little sense to Ray's daughter and moreover, they almost didn't matter. What I thought she was *really* asking for had little to do with the internal or external contributors to his rapidly declining condition and everything to do with the trust she was hesitantly placing in a world that exudes certitude, wisdom, and deep experience. My team never truly understood why he was getting worse, despite discovering his blood clot and heart problems. A few days later, I transferred him to the intensive care unit, where my jurisdiction as his doctor ended. I followed his chart in the electronic medical record, because I had hoped that his time in the ICU, with its highly methodical and scientific approach to understanding illness at the organ-system level, would be clarifying. Instead, I read about his death in his chart, and all I could glean was that his life was never really in our hands to save. I would revisit this blind alley many times in my residency.

As I was walking home the week after his death, I was surprised to run into his daughter, who waved me down and thanked me for taking care of her father. It took me a few seconds of conversation to remember who she was outside of the hospital, on the streets of our neighborhood. I was doubly surprised that she asked me to attend his funeral service at a church near my home in Harlem. She expressed her thanks for our professionalism and kindness in the care of her father. I thought back to the few times we had spoken at his bedside, where I appeared to listen intently as concern for my other patients grew by the moment. I had listened closely enough to isolate and translate clinically relevant details, but nodded through the rest. In our brief conversations, she was describing what she felt had gone wrong in a format that our healthcare system would not parse.

HOW WE MOVE FORWARD

In 2007, University of California professor Steven A. Schroeder delivered the 117th Shattuck Lecture entitled "Improving the Health of the American People" where he stated, "Health is influenced by factors in five domains— genetics, social circumstances, environmental exposures, behavioral patterns, and health care. When it comes to reducing early deaths, medical care has a relatively minor role."[23] He enjoined us doctors-in-training to more carefully consider the behavioral causes of poor health, as well as the composite "of income, total wealth, education, employment, and residential neighborhood." But the view of a clinical trainee is akin to standing at the bow of a swiftly moving ship, constitutionally forward-looking as the record of its path all but dissipates into the past, obscuring routes not taken. Today, the ship of clinical medicine is moving rapidly into genomics and personalized treatment, veering further away from the neighborhood not out of indifference, but in search of a reward promised by a century of investment in the science and technology of clinical care. Although Schroeder's perspective has been echoed clearly and forcefully by many of his contemporaries, every time I encountered a scenario like Ray's clinically unexplained death, my medical and scientific training environment guided me to inquire more deeply into biological and clinical system failures, rather than into his personal story or neighborhood context.

How we reimagine the architecture of our nation's healthcare systems will determine whether healthcare's focus on preventing death continues to remain in fundamental tension with the patient's focus on living in the neighborhood. In tension resides promise, albeit hidden from the inward gaze of healthcare professionals: this era of reform is our chance to help the healthcare system to dissolve its rigid walls. As Ray showed me, it is no longer viable to exist independently from the neighborhoods we serve.

Indeed, healthcare reform is visible on the streets of Harlem. On my way home from the hospital, I pass by vans and mobile clinics sponsored by insurance companies who are looking to recruit eligible clients. They know that many residents would not have online access, much less the ability to navigate the web-based state or federal healthcare insurance exchanges. My patients tell me that they feel good that they are finally insured, and I have seen firsthand how having healthcare insurance can mean a second chance at life without the worry of financial catastrophe. This fits with what early studies tell us—people who are newly covered report a sense of relief and even declines in depression when they have insurance.[24]

Of course, patients' sense of relief is not the only marker of a program's value and success, and it is too early to tell if simply prescribing healthcare access to more Americans will improve our nation's health. A team of economists from Harvard, the Massachusetts Institute of Technology, and the University of Chicago recently concluded that ED use substantially increases among the newly insured, as people try to make up for years of deferred care[25]—so it seems that the primary care relationship missing from Ray's life does not magically grow out of universal insurance coverage. Obviously, the fundamental patterns of how Americans and their physicians see healthcare do not automatically change with the passage of law.

Furthermore, it is unclear what an ideal patient even means. A University of California study indicated that satisfied patients are loyal to their physician, and they are less likely to use the ED. They also go to the hospital more, spend more on healthcare and drugs, and experience higher mortality.[26]

As physicians, as patients, and as community members, we all have a sense that something is wrong with our healthcare system. We see high costs, missed opportunities, patterns of outcomes that seem related to income or race or circumstance—but we can't quite say how. In this book, I take the approach that these outcomes are the inevitable result of a system designed in the absence of connection to the neighborhoods within which it is seated. As a result, it is difficult to even begin to address the biggest piece of the puzzle in healthcare reform: the question of *value* in healthcare, and of whether including the neighborhood changes the equation.

2

Heads in Beds

How am I accountable?
What counts?
Who counts?
Can you be counted on?
Will you credit my account?
By which accounting?
—David Stark, *The Sense of Dissonance:*
Accounts of Worth in Economic Life

SIX CENTS ON THE DOLLAR

A few months after Ray's death, in 2011, I finished my abridged internship and began my first teaching semester as an assistant professor of International and Public Affairs at Columbia University. I had spent the previous eight years completing my MD, PhD, and a postdoctoral fellowship in sustainable development in low-income countries. Before residency, I had spent months in rural settings spread over a dozen countries, ranging from my childhood home of Kenya to postconflict East Timor, including countries that seemed to contain dozens of countries within them, like Nigeria and India. Whenever I went to a new place with poor health outcomes, I did the same thing: I met the leaders of the region's major hospitals, I had them introduce me to the small community clinic staff in more rural areas, and then I found a community health worker to take me along on his or her daily visits to the neighborhoods and homes where people live. The community health workers introduced me to leaders of local schools, microfinance institutions, major employers (if any), and faith-based leaders, and they also showed me where and how people obtained food. It was always eye

33

opening. For instance, in southern Uganda, bananas are a major source of food and trade; farmers would take their best bananas to be turned into oil or whiskey, while leaving less nutritious bananas for themselves and their children, who were often protein-deficient and malnourished. Families who subsisted on what they grew felt like they had no other choice.[1]

I would regularly go back to the regional or national capital to work with policy makers and health-financing experts, most of whom were too busy to spend time "in the field." In most of the settings where I worked, individual healthcare was overseen and resourced by the nation or region's ministry of health, which supervised a diverse portfolio ranging from installing latrines to supporting financial cooperatives for community health workers. In most countries where budgets are constrained, healthcare delivery is an integral but proportional part of a national public health system. In countries like India or Kenya, select private hospitals augment these systems with excellent care, but they serve a fraction of the nation's population; most are compelling curios of market innovation without broad reach.

Upon my return and completion of medical school, I was granted permission by the American Board of Internal Medicine to modify my clinical training so I could translate insights from community-based health systems abroad to challenges we faced in American neighborhoods. The American healthcare system is financed both privately and publicly, at near parity, but delivered almost exclusively by hospitals that do not identify as being "government" hospitals (the Veterans Administration system is one clear exception). Even though the US Department of Health and Human Services (HHS) (1979–present) has historic roots as the Department of Health, Education, and Welfare (1953–1979), it has become increasingly focused on steering the complex healthcare sector to the exclusion of its more integrated historic mission; simultaneously, the healthcare sector has grown vastly out of proportion to the HHS department's broader public health mission.[2] Perhaps not coincidentally, we have become accustomed to hospital and clinic-based healthcare as separate and distinct from public health or local development. At Ray's funeral, I felt overwhelmed by the belief that my neighbors would eventually come to the hospital in tragic states of health that could have been avoided. And yet life in Harlem felt as distant to the hospital as the rural places I had visited from capital cities abroad. I had a notion to combine what I had learned from those community health systems[3] with homegrown concepts like Harold Freeman's patient navigators.[4]

But in order to go about this, I would first need to gauge the level of interest in such an endeavor on the part of both the hospital sector and the neighborhood. So I followed the same strategy I had used successfully abroad: I met with healthcare leaders across New York, while continuing to build relationships in Harlem.

On a cold day in early 2012, a few months after Ray had died, I arrived early to one of these meetings at Mount Sinai Hospital. I had invited Jeffrey Sachs, a prominent macroeconomist (also my postdoctoral mentor), to join me. In my view at the time, the strong presence of neighborhood community health centers, the historic origins of the patient navigator program, and insights from the Project HEED group all signaled that a locally hired health coach who bridged the neighborhood and clinic would be welcomed. After hearing me out, the administrator seemed unimpressed, and he curtly asked, "Do you know how much we get for every dollar we spend on Medicaid patients?"

"No," Professor Sachs and I both said.

"We lose six cents on every dollar. Do you know what would happen to this hospital if I filled all my beds with them?" He paused for effect and said, "Then you can understand why we don't need someone ginning up that sort of business."

Needless to say, Sachs and I left the meeting stunned. My neighbor, Ray, had been "that sort of business."[5] At the same time, I knew that hospitals across the city were facing extraordinary financial pressure. St. Vincent's Hospital in lower Manhattan, the primary site of care for those injured in the September 11 attacks, had recently closed after 161 years of service owing to rising costs and financial management challenges. Mount Sinai Hospital nearly went bankrupt less than 10 years prior. Even New York City's Health and Hospitals Corporation (HHC), a municipal agency that operates a network of public hospitals, including Harlem Hospital, had repeatedly faced significant cuts and threats to its survival.

Countless small physician practices were rapidly proving unsustainable, leading them to band together as independent practice associations or join larger healthcare systems. Financial survival had become a daily preoccupation. Rising popular concern for patient safety and a national movement for higher quality challenged the premise that a brand-name hospital or well-pedigreed physician automatically delivered better or even acceptable care.

On top of it all, healthcare providers like large hospitals were under pressure to invest in health information technology to make their inner workings more transparent, through the 2009 Health Information Technology for Economic and Clinical Health (HITECH) Act. Healthcare providers were being held accountable, and in response, they were raising prices where and when they could. Since growth in Medicaid and Medicare payments has been held consistently low nationwide as compared with private insurance companies, providers focused effort on negotiating with private insurance for higher reimbursement rates. As a result, healthcare systems knew it was much better to have a commercial payer taking up a bed than a publicly financed patient, or worse, someone without any form of insurance.

New York State was also buckling under its own healthcare spending—among the highest per person in the country.[6] The New York State Health Commissioner, Nirav Shah, had been working since 2011 to find savings in state Medicaid, and had sought a federal waiver to stabilize struggling hospitals and redesign how state Medicaid operated.[7] Healthcare providers watched Medicaid rates like a hawk, while aggressively advocating that the federal formula to calculate Medicare rates was flawed. The financial situation for all parties was precarious, to say the least, and hospital tensions were high as pressures to cut costs grew more and more acute.

On the ride back from Mount Sinai, Jeffrey Sachs reflected on our hospital encounter: "In my career of working with a range of industries, I have never heard a real person in a profession with a clear social imperative display such simplistic market reasoning." That particular administrator no longer works at Mount Sinai Hospital, but his words that day were on the money: the business of healthcare was in active tension with its social mission. Whereas Martin Steinberg had faced down hospital workers to defend his own conception of the hospital as a social unit, this administrator had simply defended the straightforward accounting realities of his financial balance sheet, without appealing to a higher purpose of any kind. According to Columbia sociologist Adam Reich, the anonymous administrator, embedded in a hospital with a historic social mission, gives us insight into something bigger:

> We should be looking for situations in which people try and fail to connect their values with their economic activities, for situations in which people use thin moral scripts to justify their economic activities, and for situations

in which market actors seem to generate a self-referential conception of morality—a morality of efficiency. We should be looking not only for connected lives but for contradictory lives, as individuals and organizations work imperfectly to reconcile their values with broader forces out of their control.[8]

Indeed, there are broader forces at work. Healthcare costs in New York State are absorbing a larger share of local and state budgets. This leads to underinvestment in everything that a healthier life depends upon.

Massachusetts, a state that has historically supported social programs like universal health insurance, has been witness to the social costs of rising healthcare expenditures. As healthcare leader and former gubernatorial candidate Don Berwick explains:

> Public higher education: down 26 percent. Early childhood education and care: down 28 percent. Local aid: down 44 percent. Parks and recreation: down 43 percent. Meanwhile, state health care expenditures increased 63 percent. The patterns are similar on the private side. For businesses, the state's medical costs, which are the highest in the nation, are one of the most substantial barriers to growth; and laborers' take-home pay has at best stayed level, whereas their out-of-pocket medical costs and payroll deductions for health insurance have soared.[9]

Whether progressive or conservative, we cannot escape the reality that soaring healthcare costs have posed an existential threat to the health of Americans. The logic that drives socially progressive politicians to reform public healthcare programs like Medicaid, because its growth squeezes social programs, is the same logic that impels governors of more conservative states to privatize the management of public funds and healthcare systems. New York City's own sprawling public hospital system was turned over to the Health and Hospital Corporation (HHC), a quasi-public agency, in 1969, a year after the private Hospital Corporation of America (HCA) was founded. The former has been plagued by poor quality and responsiveness, while the latter is now the largest publicly traded, for-profit operator of healthcare facilities in the world. It also has a storied history of financial fraud. The classic criticism against treating hospitals like a market enterprise is that quality of care would suffer in a rush to maximize profits. However, a Harvard group led by Ashish K. Jha found that there was no change in quality when hospitals converted from nonprofit to for-profit status, including the proportion of poor and minority patients served.[10]

In some ways, this is no surprise, since large nonprofit healthcare systems that are under financial pressure often focus on the same issues that for-profit systems do, rendering legal financial status moot.[11] But there is a difference: when the financial margins of for-profit systems do improve, the surplus goes to shareholders or equity owners, or to reinvestment and expansion activities. Nonprofit hospitals, on the other hand, are expected to maintain their tax-exempt status by reinvesting a portion of their margins into activities that benefit their communities. Unfortunately, the enforcement of this requirement is muddled and leadership-dependent.[12] Even at the nonprofit HHC, which is currently led by Ram Raju, fiscal stewardship remains a social mission: "If you are a C.E.O. and you do not collect the dollar that you are supposed to collect so that you can give services to other people, then there is a social justice issue for me . . . My incompetency cannot cost another person care."[13] In this context, the Mount Sinai ex-administrator's comments seem less surprising. Everyone I spoke to at the time seemed stuck, exhibiting the same survival instincts. Although few were as blunt as the administrator I met, most healthcare leaders were preoccupied with "mission-critical" issues, which rendered the neighborhood a distant realm.

In June 2012, while I was discouraged and struggling to understand how Ray's children and grandchildren would live a better life than he did in this context, the politics of the Patient Protection and Affordable Care Act (ACA) flooded the media. The headline premise of the ACA is best described by one of its lead architects, Harvard economist David Cutler: "The law has two overarching goals: Cover almost everyone, and slow the growth of medical care costs. Both goals are equally important. Too little coverage, and premiums in the exchanges will be unaffordable; too rapid a cost increase, and the federal government [taxpayers] will not be able to afford the subsidies."[14] Girded by the ubiquitous mantra of "bending the [growth in healthcare] cost curve," these simplifications form the theoretical basis for what the ACA is supposed to do.

For systems like HHC, the ACA's mission aligned with providing care to all New Yorkers, and for enormous companies like HCA, the ACA would increase the overall market of insured patients and contribute to cost-reduction pressures. Large systems like HHC and HCA staked out an early position amid the tidal force winds of reform, whereas smaller hospitals like Mount Sinai had to weather the rippling consequences of change while being mindful of competitors, or create stability by increasing in size and building financial reserves for the uncertain times ahead.

To understand how we got to this fevered pitch, we need to look back to the momentous period surrounding the enactment of Medicare and Medicaid as part of the Social Security Amendments of 1965 by President Lyndon B. Johnson. The legislation made healthcare financing for qualifying Americans a "mandatory" item in the federal budget,[15] as opposed to the "discretionary" spending on programs supported through annual appropriation bills—items like public education, transportation, housing, veterans benefits, or food systems.[16]

50 YEARS OF HERALDED GROWTH

In 1963, a few years before Harold Freeman arrived at Harlem Hospital and Ray shipped out to Vietnam, the influential future Nobel Prize–winning economist Kenneth J. Arrow published a seminal paper titled "Uncertainty and the Welfare Economics of Medical Care." In it, he noted that "the subject is the medical-care industry, not health. . . . A transfer of purchasing power from the well to the ill will increase the demand for medical services. This will manifest itself in the short run in an increase in the price of medical services and in the long run in an increase in the amount supplied."[17]

In his succinct introduction, Arrow anticipated what is now popularly called the "sick care industry,"[18] which places market power in the hands of the sick by focusing payments on hospitals and clinicians who diagnose and treat patients. After more than a half-century of this dynamic, a clinical diagnosis was Ray's ticket to the considerable financial and institutional resources encompassed by the health sector, which commands nearly a fifth of the US gross domestic product (GDP) with $3 trillion of activity.[19] When he went to the ER, Ray found that highly skilled physicians were suddenly there for him. These professionals comprise a formidable industry in their own right (3.6 percent of GDP),[20] only second in the entire economy to hospital services (5.6 percent of GDP), ahead of construction, agriculture, automobile, and technology industries. For the most part, modern healthcare systems operate as their underlying financial architecture would suggest. In practical terms, Ray was not a healthcare consumer until he became sick, and as he became sicker, more resources were deployed and consumed until he died.

Arrow postulated that healthcare has significant features and purposes that differentiate it from a traditional market-based sector. He states, "when the market fails to achieve an optimal state, society will, to some extent at least, recognize the gap, and non-market social institutions will arise attempting to bridge it."[21] In his paper, he succinctly anticipated the consequence of making medical care the focus of the overall health equation: it would dominate over time. This part seems spot on, as the average American family of four is now paying over $23,000 per year for medical care alone.[22] In fact, a decade of wage increases for the same family of four has been wiped out by growth in healthcare costs, leaving us less free to invest in all the other ingredients we know are crucial to living healthy lives.[23] As Charles Roehrig of the Altarum Institute put it, we have "a triangle of painful choices"[24] ahead as we choose between healthcare spending, everything else in the economy, or increasing total revenue from tax increases in a divisive political climate. Decreasing healthcare spending is not something regulators can simply turn the dial to achieve. The choices for a nation faced with financing healthcare for an unprecedented number of individuals, including a bulge of baby boomers who will be eligible for Medicare, seem stark: less of everything else or more taxes.

When I keep this dynamic in mind, it becomes possible to imagine being part of a growing healthcare sector that continually gets more efficient at treating illness, while the people in my neighborhood have fewer opportunities to proactively stay healthy and build wealth. Instead, they get sicker and poorer over time. Although the healthcare system receives the lion's share of credit for improvements in the health of Americans, it actually hits well below its $3 trillion weight across many measures. What we are left with is a sector that performs a limited subset of what it takes to keep America healthy. Public health experts and community development practitioners have been sounding an alarm for decades. The struggle to transform a healthcare sector is national in scope and beyond the control of any particular group of people or networks. Few disagree with the premise that the healthcare sector needs to change.

In late 2012, two months after an ACA-related penalty for hospital readmissions was implemented, I was contacted by another group at Mount

Sinai. Their newly formed readmissions team (Preventable Admissions Care Team or PACT), a nationally recognized program that uses a data-driven and sociological lens for patient care, wanted to learn about community health workers (CHWs).[25] As winter progressed, I heard from a few other New York City hospitals that had initially shown little interest in adding a CHW layer to their system. A small group of healthcare leaders, emerging from large healthcare systems with historic social missions, were among the first to recognize that upheaval could also be an opportunity.

HIGH-VALUE HEALTHCARE

In 2013, Steven Brill published a gripping 24,000-word polemic in *Time*. I heard about "The Bitter Pill" from my parents, who had heard about it from their neighbors in Indianapolis. Upheaval began to permeate every aspect of healthcare delivery and consumption. People were paying attention and they wanted answers.

But to what end?

The *charge master*, an ominously named roster of secretive and highly variable hospital list prices, was the object of villainy in Brill's piece. By choosing it, he shifted (or extended) historic patient anger from insurance companies to healthcare systems. Arguing back, healthcare systems stated that the charge master was a red herring, and that prices are negotiated with private insurers to levels that rarely approach the list price. Public interest advocates argued that the uninsured pay the inflated prices, to which hospitals responded that they are rarely able to collect upon this "uncompensated care."

With an estimated $700 billion of waste in the healthcare sector,[26] there is good reason to take a closer look. Clear answers are rarely forthcoming: the circular arguments remind me of Bill Keane's *Family Circus* cartoons, where Jeffy wanders a jungle in his dreams, tracing out a random path that leads him back to where he started; the jungle is the American healthcare sector. Like many readers, I concluded that Brill was speaking to *me*, as a discerning consumer who should ask, just as Brill did, if I'm getting my money's worth for my healthcare.

This question can be turned into an ideal frame for the long-standing debates about value in healthcare. The same year that the ACA was passed—and a year before Brill posed the question for a mass readership—Harvard Business School's Michael Porter proposed a paradigm shift for the question of value in a seminal *New England Journal of Medicine* article:

> Achieving high value for patients must become the overarching goal of health care delivery, with **value defined as the health outcomes achieved per dollar spent.** This goal is what matters for patients and unites the interests of all actors in the system. If value improves, patients, payers, providers, and suppliers can all benefit while the economic sustainability of the health care system increases. . . . Current cost-measurement approaches have also obscured value in health care and led to cost-containment efforts that are incremental, ineffective, and sometimes even counterproductive. Today, health care organizations measure and accumulate costs around departments, physician specialties, discrete service areas, and line items such as drugs and supplies—a reflection of the organization and financing of care. Costs, like outcomes, should instead be measured around the patient. [my emphasis][27]

Porter's concept of value is both expansive and simple. Taken in its most open-ended form, it is possible that the path to achieving better health outcomes—via better education, higher income, a safer street or block, deeper social support systems—may not even reside within the reach of healthcare systems. However, since there *are* clear avenues to improve efficiencies within and across healthcare systems, focusing upon traditional healthcare sector actors as the drivers of higher value has emerged as a nearly unarguable point of consensus. To date, value has been defined in slippery ways, leading to "divergent approaches, gaming of the system, and slow progress in performance improvement."[28] For instance, the American Medical Association, a historically powerful physician lobby group, plays an influential role in rate setting for individual services through the Relative Value Update Committee (RUC). It is comprised largely of anonymous specialists nominated by associations, and their recommendations are nearly always (as in 90 percent of the time) accepted by the Centers for Medicare and Medicaid Services.[29] Of course, there are no representatives that primarily hold patient, consumer, or citizen perspectives. Primary care doctors are in the minority on the RUC; accordingly, most preventative and primary care measures—a simple test, verbal counseling, or nonclinical support—are reimbursed poorly. In other words, thanks to the RUC, primary care is treated as a low-value part of the healthcare system.

In Porter's assessment, however, the work of the primary care doctor, if she can demonstrate longitudinal improvements in the health outcomes of her patients, should be seen as high value. Furthermore, Porter's value-based system has the capacity to flip tensions that segregate, into forces for collaboration: "For any condition or population, multiple outcomes collectively define success."[30] By extension, efforts to improve education, income, street safety, and social support services could be seen as integral to a healthcare system's success.

Porter's arguments are a fresh riff on an old argument about what constitutes a good use of money in healthcare: *let's move from doing more healthcare (volume) to doing what leads to better health outcomes (value)*. The possibility of calculating better health outcomes based upon objective data, spreading the financial risk across a population, and simultaneously defining who is accountable for care allowed the ACA to survive in an adversarial political environment.

FROM VOLUME TO VALUE

The search for value as defined by Porter has the potential to align large-scale health objectives with the concerns of healthcare consumers regardless of where they live in America. This is important as the ACA's legislative tendrils lose their fragile coherence when unfurled across 50 states, 3,643 hospital service areas,[31] and approximately 200,000[32] American neighborhoods. In *Reinventing American Health Care*, senior ACA advisor Ezekiel Emmanuel provides an insider view of how the demands of hospitals, physician groups, insurance companies, pharmaceutical companies, and powerful lobbying interests were balanced and appeased to get the bill through. One of the ACA's lead economists even suggested that writing obscure legislation would be the only way to have it pass, exploiting the "stupidity of the American voter."[33] Mantras like *volume to value* easily outlive the nuances of law.

As an academic and a physician, I feel at sea whenever friends ask me for an authoritative "thumbs up or down" about the ACA—it is hard to know what anyone is talking about when they refer to it. Most of my neighbors in Harlem see the ACA as a civil rights issue and a way to support the embattled president. In my parents' home state of Indiana, the ACA is seen as a heavy-handed encroachment on individual liberties and state rights.[34] How Americans feel about the ACA, now that it has survived multiple legislative and legal challenges, is informed by both political preference and personal experience: whether the ACA gave them access to expanded coverage, whether they got a better or worse deal, whether they got to continue with their favorite healthcare providers, and whether they could navigate the clumsy rollout of the federal and state insurance Internet-based exchanges. I still cannot see how Ray's remaining family will live fundamentally better lives as a direct result of the ACA or how their health will improve. They already had access to multiple nearby hospital systems, which they entered when absolutely necessary. When they needed to be seen at a clinic or hospital, they always had some form of insurance, like most Americans even before the ACA.[35] On the hospital side, an expanded current and future market of insured consumers promises a lucrative business for healthcare systems that can figure out a viable path forward through the new labyrinth of reimbursements and conditions of payment attached to state Medicaid and federal Medicare. Those hospital systems and insurance companies that cannot adapt are going belly-up or being acquired.

The result is a mix of mergers, acquisitions, and alliances as healthcare systems increase in size and scale in the name of efficiency, access more financing, and seek greater market share. For example, in 2013, Mount Sinai Hospital became the flagship facility of the largest healthcare system in New York City by merging with Continuum Health Partners; it now operates in more than 200 neighborhoods across the city.[36]

Still, it is difficult to separate the effects of the ACA from long-time-coming industry trends; hospitals were closing and merging in droves well before ACA passage. Moreover, a healthcare system with footprints in hundreds of neighborhoods does not necessarily lead to better health outcomes within them. The ACA explicitly creates avenues to better health outside the walls of the hospital, but these are only visible to those willing to parse its obscure language. It is akin to a Swiss army knife: if you carefully examine its dozens of provisions, you will find opportunities for healthcare systems to systematically redesign their relationships with the different communities within the neighborhoods they serve.

Two seemingly separate ACA concepts—"Accountable Care Organization (ACO)" and "readmission penalties"—have proven effective in expanding the scope of healthcare system activity out of the hospital. The ACO concept was shepherded by the Center for Medicare and Medicaid Innovations (CMMI) Center, established in 2011 by an ACA provision with a budget providing $10 billion for 10 years. The concept of an accountable care organization was originally coined by Elliott Fisher, director of the Dartmouth Institute for Health Policy and Clinical Practice, and initially developed with the support of Mark McClellan, who led the Value Initiative at Brookings Institution. The ACO concept rewires the logic of financial payments from one where individual clinicians (and their hospitals) received volume-based fees for services provided, to one in which clinicians receive a monthly sum to provide all care for a set population of patients, linked to performance improvement over time. Bypassing the RUC, the ACO allowed healthcare systems to test new models of care at their own financial risk, discover savings through higher-value activities, and invest in smarter care delivery systems if they were successful. One such model of care is the Patient Centered Medical Home (PCMH), which aims to consolidate a patient's many interactions with the healthcare system around a core of primary care. Perhaps most importantly, healthcare providers who adopted some form of ACO model, even for just a subset of their patients, found a network of peers working on the same effort across the country. Collaborative networks that advanced collective learning formed, and fences between healthcare systems began to lower as they faced a common challenge. Ironically, the administrator I encountered above was tasked with establishing an ACO for Mount Sinai. The shift in mindset it required was significant, and the individual moved on.

The second ACA instrument, "readmission penalties," reflects a change in the conditions of how payments flow to hospitals from Medicare. At many hospitals nationwide, like Mount Sinai, a large fraction of patients who received treatment would quickly return (as "readmissions"). Some of the most common reasons for readmissions include misunderstandings about a diagnosis, confusion about medications, poor social support at home, and lack of follow-up appointments.[37] The new rule penalizes all hospitals that readmit a greater fraction of their patients than what the Centers for Medicare and Medicaid Services defines as allowable. Initially, healthcare systems with patients in tough neighborhoods pushed back against the readmissions penalty policy, citing forces outside hospital control as the chief culprits of excessive readmissions; Mount Sinai Health System CEO Kenneth Davis was among them:

Fragile or absent in many communities are reliable transportation services, quality housing, flexible child or elder care assistance, and relevant job training … Improving population health and reducing hospitalizations— especially high rates of readmissions—are everyone's goals, but hospitals can only provide part of the solution. In order to lower costs, we need to invest in social support services outside of our health care institutions.[38]

Davis and many other healthcare leaders across the country, including leading academics, offered well-reasoned arguments that readmission penalties should be adjusted for socioeconomic status of the patient population under specific conditions.[39] The penalties have been implemented uniformly and readmission rates have decreased nationwide,[40] despite evidence that the penalty is regressive.[41] With their hands forced, hospitals had to seriously consider what happened when patients got home, particularly if they did not have a home to go to. Guidelines were put in place and a follow-up system was developed to ensure that patients did not bounce back to the hospital after their discharge to the neighborhood. Health improvement outside the hospital suddenly had value inside the hospital all the way up the administrative food chain.

As a result, those healthcare professionals who had always been concerned about the hospital's social mission—like Project HEED and Health Leads—now had the pretext to build on their work. For example, Mount Sinai Health System's readmissions program, PACT, was put on a fast track for expansion. And information sharing among institutions acquired increased significance. Health information exchanges between hospitals are touted as important means of sharing information about a patient who is bouncing between facilities. Summing up these changes in *Forbes* magazine, Davis wrote:

The hospital of today is a stand-alone facility where services are provided mostly within its walls, and quality of care is too often measured by number of inpatient beds. The number of inpatient beds in a hospital does not equate to better care in a community. This is an outdated metric, particularly in an era where numerous specialties, including pediatrics and HIV/AIDS, require mostly outpatient treatment. The hospital of tomorrow needs to be a large, integrated system providing extensive outpatient care beyond its primary facility, dedicated to keeping community members healthy. A well-cared-for population should require less inpatient care, leading to lower demand for hospital beds.[42]

A healthcare system that shares this vision needs to change its architecture to transform its presence beyond the walls of a healthcare facility. But it is unclear how much. Instead of waiting for Ray to get sick as he bounced around across neighborhood hospitals, the healthcare system of the future that Davis envisions would actively monitor his health and collaborate with him to ensure his well-being. It is a compelling vision. However, most healthcare system operations, financial assets, and information systems are completely disconnected from the support people need outside a clinical network.

Economists today are on the fence about what a new era of large, integrated healthcare systems means for prices, costs, performance, innovation, or outcomes. Just as a ubiquitous healthcare system does not in and of itself yield better health outcomes, simply saying that we are moving in the direction of higher value does not make it so. The Federal Trade Commission and Department of Justice are all watching closely to discern if the consequence of bigger, more dominant systems is higher costs than the expected norm.[43] However, it is difficult to gauge what constitutes normal fluctuations versus trends that intensify the triangle of painful choices that Roehrig described. The insatiable beast of healthcare costs is being rapidly shifted to the consumer.

The big questions that grip the management of healthcare systems have become only more difficult to explain to outsiders, and even well-reported popular articles like Brill's in *Time* do not provide entrée to the discussions that truly shape healthcare. Americans are still outsiders, and now, more than ever, healthcare systems need their participation—even, I would argue, their guidance.

HEALTHCARE MOVES INTO THE NEIGHBORHOOD

The paucity of constructive external guidance leaves the healthcare system of the new era with a vexing problem. The mega-networks in New York City, for example, cannot afford to wait until the factors that drive disease—individual choices and contextual circumstances—progress to the point where a person acquires a disease diagnosis. At the same time, they are constrained by evidence-based guidelines, financial analyses, information systems, and operational protocols in their efforts to bring the *right people*, at the *right time*, into the *right part of the healthcare system*. Especially when the right parts and truly proactive strategies don't yet exist. Wrong movements and misdirected energy result in enormous waste on all sides and put people in danger. Since healthcare systems do not possess the experience, primary mandate, or the relationships to address the major factors that push people toward chronic medical conditions and early death—such issues as low income and insufficient education—they do not yet have the wherewithal to pull off their new responsibilities safely and effectively.

Imagine that a 25-year-old version of Ray had come to see me, a primary care doctor, in 2014, two years after the ACA rollout. First of all, it would have been unusual, because his health, like that of most young men, would have been relatively normal, as measured by the healthcare system, and few young men bother to go to the doctor when they feel well.

My questions about his nutrition and diet would have been minimal. Even if I had checked on markers of diabetes or heart disease—perhaps because he had a strong family history of both—they would have likely been normal. If he smoked, I would have assessed his motivation to quit, and calibrated my approach to his own goals. It is unlikely I would have asked him about his job prospects, because there would be little I could do about employment, despite knowing that a satisfying job would be some of the best medicine he could have. Years later, if he came back, I might have noted that he was getting heavier, and because some preventive care is covered by the ACA, it is likely that I would have tested him for early signs of diabetes. If he were pre-diabetic, I would have referred him to the YMCA's diabetes prevention program, even though there was no obvious way for us to jointly support him in a coordinated fashion. In so doing, we may have delayed the onset of diabetes by a few years. As a senior he would have been enrolled in an ACO program that finally gave him the comprehensive diabetes care he needed.

If his wife died before he did, it is possible that a care coordinator or social worker would have noted her passing; however, it is unlikely that he would have been offered extra support for "normal grieving." Having lost a pillar of his universe, his decline could still ensue. In this imaginary scenario, however, his readmissions would be carefully monitored and I am sure that the costs related to his end-of-life care would be better contained. Because of the dogged advocacy of palliative care pioneers, at some point we would have sat down with him and his daughter to understand his goals and aims as he lived out the remaining days of his life. Instead of dying in the ICU, a better outcome for him, his family, and the healthcare system would have been dying at home among friends and family, the setting a majority of Americans desire. Is this scenario better than what he experienced? Yes.

Is this the best we can do? Not even close.

MUTUAL INFORMATION, DIFFERENT CONCLUSIONS

Today, healthcare leaders have to reconsider the practical implications of a system that resembles a starburst with hospitals at the center of an extensive network of outpatient care settings that lie in wait for patients to fall into their web. The HITECH Act, as flat-footed as it has been in subsidizing the growth of clunky information systems, has definitely made information a powerful currency and motivator for healthcare improvement, on par with financing. It is more possible today than in Ray's era to use healthcare information to discover better ways to invest healthcare dollars than in traditional clinical services.

The records of our lives embedded in healthcare data also reflect the powerful influence of social and economic factors—education or the lack thereof, opportunity or exploitation, spiritual support and mental stress—as well as the biological basis of disease. Seen this way, it is our responsibility as neighbors to impel healthcare systems to be an active force in informing how a healthier life is assembled in relevant contexts. I am confident that when opportunities to integrate health and social services are framed clearly, in a data-driven and financially clear manner, healthcare leaders will build bridges into the neighborhood where it aligns with their evolving mission. I am less confident that those with a street-level view will consider the demanding requirements of interacting with healthcare systems to be a valuable use of their time. However, without their perspective, it seems inevitable that the high-value healthcare system of the future will inadvertently (or purposely) cherry-pick the patients who are already in the best position to receive healthcare according to existing system designs.

Healthcare systems cannot collaborate with what they cannot or choose not to see. Today, our community-based groups and neighborhood establishments are virtually invisible to the vertically integrated world of healthcare

systems. There is no common point of control among neighborhood organizations, no definitive body of methods and practices for collective action.
Very few of these groups organize their members into strong professions
that advocate for their own interests. In my work with community health
workers abroad, I saw their powerful effect on healthcare professionals as
they revealed local infrastructures that contribute to a population's health.
In contrast to the shifting abstraction of a healthcare-centric "population,"
the neighborhood has a finite geographic area with social and political
dynamics largely independent of the workings and logic of adjacent healthcare systems. As a result, the meaning of *high-value* healthcare changes
considerably when the neighborhood and healthcare systems share mutual
information about their capabilities and aims.

Without a deeper understanding of the neighborhood, our nation is in
danger of spending extraordinary amounts of money and energy spinning
its wheels in an effort to transform to a modern healthcare system.

3

A Purposeful Neighborhood

What is a system? A system is a network of interdependent components that work together to try to accomplish the aim of the system. A system must have an aim. Without an aim, there is no system. The aim of the system must be clear to everyone in the system. The aim must include plans for the future. The aim is a value judgment.
—W. Edwards Deming

THE AIM OF A NEIGHBORHOOD

What is a neighborhood? Does it exist within a certain block, within certain institutions—schools, churches, corner stores—within those streets, within a certain group of people? Are its boundaries set by street numbers, or by the whereabouts of its inhabitants? None of these criteria quite fit—no two people may agree on precisely what defines any one neighborhood.

The study of systems theory gives us a more flexible language with which to describe and understand neighborhoods. As explained by W. Edwards Deming, "a system is a network of interdependent components that work together to try to accomplish the aim of the system."[1] In this language, we might understand that every individual assembles his own neighborhood—his own network of interdependent people, places, and institutions—that works toward the aim of a healthier, happier, fuller life for that individual. That is not to say that no two neighborhoods overlap or are even the same: a person living on 125th and Park and a person on 126th and Lexington will both identify their neighborhood as East Harlem and, if pressed, will describe many of the same locations, institutions, and people as being part of it. Ultimately what matters is not whether these systems match exactly, but how each person locates himself within his system, his neighborhood.

51

By centering the neighborhood on the individual, and understanding it not as a static place but as a dynamic and purposeful system, we can begin to understand the ways in which neighborhoods interact with health.

Years ago, the medical sociologist Aaron Antonovsky proposed a relationship between stress, health, and well-being to explain why some people thrive and others struggle in times of stress. The people who thrive, he said, have a "'sense of coherence,' the ability to understand the situation they are in, have reasons to improve their health and have the power and resources—material, social or psychological—to cope with stress and challenges."[2] He called this a salutogenic ("health creating") model, which is correlated to other measures of quality of life. While the methods medical students and residents learn can sharply define a problem or disparity and allow us to recognize what is unhealthy in a person or a place, the salutogenic model focuses on the resources and capacities that people have to impact their health—in other words, their neighborhood. These are complementary concepts, but today, they stand as far apart as a hospital floor and a town hall meeting.

RAY'S BLOCK

According to his daughter, Ray did not feel safe where he lived. When I walk on the streets near his building, I can empathize with him. Not too far from his apartment is the express subway stop of the 4/5/6 train that thousands of people use every day to travel to and from Harlem. It is a bustling corner, a dilute remnant of what Harlem must have been like in the 1980s and 1990s: emaciated addicts and early morning drunks amidst people who are moving from their second to third jobs or headed downtown to their offices. One-dollar pizza stores are in high production early in the morning, and the Pathmark grocery store across the street is a haven for loiterers. Every morning, homeless shelters from across the region drop people off at this corner, next door to the highest concentration of methadone clinics in the city. But Ray was just another old-timer on the block, subject to the daily hustle. Seniors in the area state the same thing: they can't just go outside for a walk on their intimidating block.[3] Even the occasional presence of cops does not make them feel safe—often, quite the contrary.

I never gave much thought to why this block, in particular, feels particularly unsafe, until I got to know Clyde Williams. I met Williams while he was running for the congressional seat of Harlem's legendary 23-term congressman, Charles "Charlie" Rangel, in 2012. I admired Williams because, even though he lost his bid, he followed through on conversations he had had with my neighbors. Williams and his wife, Mona Stuphen, weren't new to politics—they met while working in the White House, and Williams quickly became involved in local politics when they left DC. He struck up a particularly good relationship with seniors, who liked his straightforward manner and hardscrabble southern roots.

At the Casabe House, a historic senior center not far from where Ray lived, we both heard complaint after complaint about methadone clinics, which seniors saw as the source of the problem. Methadone is basically an analog of heroin. It blocks the feeling of withdrawal that addicts experience as they try to quit and doesn't give the user the same high. The idea is to start methadone maintenance therapy and then slowly taper it down. The truth is that most people stay on methadone for life, coming to the clinics on a daily basis for decades.

As a physician, I've always seen methadone clinics as an ally in healthcare. They help people step down from the ravages of heroin addiction, strictly monitor clients for other drug abuse, and keep careful track of the methadone itself, lest it be sold illegally on the streets. It is not a perfect solution, but it is one of the few options out there to help deal with a national epidemic that hits places like Harlem as well as rural towns and suburban neighborhoods in well-to-do areas. They are also a source of perennial complaint from neighbors who fear violence or drug dealing from the clinic's clientele, making them targets for "not in my backyard" campaigns. So where do they go? They gravitate toward neighborhoods that do not have the power or influence to keep them out. To put this in context, 30 percent of methadone clinics in Manhattan are in one neighborhood, East Harlem, and there are eight clinics in one building, right near the subway stop and senior center. Why were so many of the methadone clinics disproportionately in one block in one neighborhood, particularly when the people they serve come from all over the city?

For years Ray simply stayed indoors whenever he could. We can't know exactly why, but his daughter spoke about his deep disappointment with how Harlem was turning out in the decades since he had returned from Vietnam. His sedentary lifestyle primed him for every chronic condition he was at risk for, and accelerated the conditions when they arrived. The walkability of a neighborhood has an indirect impact on local health. If the key to preventing or managing diabetes is diet, exercise, and medication when necessary, it is fair to say that Ray started out behind the curve. Williams heard from seniors who were in similar circumstances when he visited with Casabe House residents.

In 2014, after a woman was stabbed to death outside of a clinic near the subway stop, Williams decided to take action. He saw the concentration of these clinics in a low-income, predominantly minority part of the neighborhood as a civil rights violation, whereas I, a physician-in-training, had simply thought about them as improving access to care. After Ray's death, I knew it was my view that needed the adjustment: the microcosm of this block is a window into how the health of a neighborhood is shaped by forces that are decades and even centuries in the making. Those forces had a direct impact on the assets available for individuals like Ray to assemble toward the purpose of a healthier life.

"LOCATION, LOCATION, LOCATION"

In 1776, the Battle of Harlem Heights raged between the outnumbered Continental Army, led by Gen. George Washington and the well-equipped British Army. General Washington earned his first victory, boosting the morale of the fledgling army that would forge a new republic. Famous settlers, such as Alexander Hamilton, owned fertile agricultural land in Harlem until nutrients were stripped and property sold. After the Panic of 1873 led to a marked drop in property values, the City of New York assimilated the boom-and-bust village of Harlem. Waves of Irish, Italian, and Jewish immigrants populated the area, particularly East Harlem, and by 1876 numerous tenements had been erected to accommodate the growing population.[4] Gas pipes were installed in anticipation of rapid development of the area. An 1893 edition of *Harlem Monthly Magazine* described the spirit of the neighborhood at the time: "it is evident to the most superficial observer that the centre of fashion, wealth, culture, and intelligence, must, in the near future, be found in the ancient and honorable village of Harlem."

By the middle of the twentieth century, the "ancient village" of Harlem had segmented into Columbia University–dominated Morningside Heights, African American Central Harlem, and a largely Puerto Rican East Harlem. It also included parts of Hamilton and Washington Heights, the latter extended north into a largely Dominican enclave. The Great Migration of African Americans at the turn of the century from segregationist southern states had brought nearly 100,000 African Americans to Central Harlem. White families living in Harlem left by the tens of thousands; some organized and implemented discriminatory housing patterns that bled the meager wealth of newcomers. Around the same time, Puerto Ricans began arriving in East Harlem in unprecedented numbers, searching for jobs as the government launched "Operation Bootstrap" to industrialize Manhattan and transfer Puerto Rican assets to corporations. Mayor Robert Wagner campaigned to increase the Puerto Rican population in order to fill factory jobs, and East Harlem went from being known as Italian Harlem, Negro Harlem, and Spanish Harlem to simply *El Barrio* ("the neighborhood"), reflecting the dominant presence of Spanish speakers.[5] The number of bodegas increased with the new population and the now-dormant La Marqueta hosted hundreds of vendors.

As these newcomers arrived, the Jewish population, which numbered 200,000 in 1915, dwindled to 5,000 by 1930, leaving Mount Sinai Hospital on the border of a rapidly changing neighborhood. Italians took their leave later in the century, steadied longer by the informal power of the infamous Mafioso as well as talented politicians who were able to win the support of other ethnic groups, exemplified by Fiorello H. La Guardia. By 1946, however, a *Time* article spoke derogatively about the neighborhood's reputation and worried about new political forces at work in its midst: "The core of Manhattan's sprawling 18th Congressional District is a verminous, crime-ridden slum called East Harlem. Its hordes of Italians, Puerto Ricans, Jews and Negroes have traditionally voted Republican. But in the last decade a new force came into power: the patchwork patronage machine of shrill, stooped, angry-eyed, pro-Communist Representative Vito Marcantonio."[6]

The neighborhood was bursting at the seams with a shifting array of people by the time Ray was a young resident. Tension between landlords and renters grew as conditions deteriorated. East Harlem was deemed a slum and the neighborhood was "redlined," a discriminatory practice where investment and services slowed to a trickle, accelerating already poor conditions. People organized and renters fought back. Politicians like Marcantonio worked closely with the East Harlem community to bring a small number of new housing projects to the neighborhood, which were largely well received. Despite the growing discontent, trust among neighbors remained:

Growing up in East Harlem we didn't have window bars. And if your neighbor needed a cup of coffee, they knocked on the door and took whatever
they wanted and they would say, "I took a bottle of milk and I owe you a bottle of milk." And people trusted each other in those days. We were not poor,
but we were rich in our own way and each family had the same thing, and
everyone had a lot and a little. What each family had, we all shared and it
was very family oriented. Every family was like your own family and that's
the way it was back then.[7]

The streets of East Harlem were a place for stickball, shaved ice, group par-
enting, and small businesses, so long as you stayed near your block.

In 1951, when Ray was a boy, the New York City Housing Authority
wanted to condemn tenements across more than 150 acres of city-owned
land to provide space for new buildings. The city agreed, and hundreds of
buildings and businesses were razed to make way for superblocks inspired
by the famed architect Le Corbusier, who had excited urban planners and
politicians with his vision of "towers in a park" to reduce congestion, "un-
slum" neighborhoods, and manage pollution. Ray's family moved into one
of these buildings from their home in Central Harlem, along with 75,000
others at the cost of over $300 million.[8]

In her famously defiant book, *The Death and Life of Great American Cities*, Jane Jacobs excoriated established architects, urban planners, and bu-
reaucrats for destroying the vibrant life of urban neighborhoods across
America, replacing it with dour standardization. She was moved to write
by her cursory familiarity with East Harlem.[9] By 1956, more than 1,500
businesses were lost, along with thousands of jobs, many never to be replaced. The blow to the social fabric of the neighborhood was devastating.
Bureaucratic processes and self-selection led to greater racial segregation,
giving way to a generation of racially aligned politics at a time of growing
civil rights struggle. Politicians like Marcantonio, who were elected with
the support of a diverse population, have yet to make a comeback. Central
Harlem became a major epicenter of the national African American civil
rights movement, whereas East Harlem's Puerto Rican self-determination
movement became peripheral. Despite what appeared to be a higher level
of political cohesion to achieve the goals of specific groups, the street-level
social fabric was falling apart.

Economic transformation followed physical transformation: unemployment soared as families were dislocated, social networks disrupted, businesses shuttered, and the requirements of low-income housing kept the neighborhood poor by definition. The Johnson administration unveiled the Great Society programs when Ray was a teenager, and 50 years later, nearly all of the surviving programs are still heavily used in East Harlem. Economists like Columbia University's Douglas Almond have shown that many of these safety-net programs have reduced obesity and diabetes in children while improving the economic self-sufficiency of women.[10] However, federal programs associated with the Department of Housing and Urban Development (HUD) historically relied upon central administrative control, creating distance from the neighborhood, breeding discontent, and generating new forms of bureaucratic complexity. A 1967 issue of *Life* magazine quoted the leader of a group that called themselves the *Real* Great Society: "We knew President Johnson was trying to get to us, but he just didn't know how. He just never in the groove, man." Another member elaborated, "He just didn't have our background . . . You don't just change your role and come on as a savior."[11]

By the 1970s, a number of neighborhood organizations like Union Settlement Association rose in prominence as hubs of trusted health and social services.[12] However, even with the help of public financing, local organizations could barely steady the devastation to the neighborhood's social fabric, what the Columbia psychiatrist Mindy Fullilove calls "root shock." The street-level dynamism of the neighborhood shifted underground, and informal gangs, businesses, and community-based organizations tried to bridge the paradoxical lack of opportunity amidst a maze of services. Drugs flooded in and crime skyrocketed in a pattern that would continue through the 1990s.[13] Famous musicians like Tupac Shakur and Marc Anthony were born in these challenging environs, but the significant artistic, literary, and cultural achievements of residents were largely overshadowed by East Harlem's reputation as a seedy underbelly of Manhattan.

David Erickson, an urban historian, wrote about the cataclysmic national impact of housing programs:

> In a seminal [1973] report, the Ford Foundation put much of the blame
> for federal housing policy failures on HUD's partners. Ford's criticism was
> that an influx of resources from the federal level overwhelmed local governments and other institutions. The report concluded that "the mismatch

between society's capacity to provide resources and the limited ability of local communities to absorb and use them effectively" was responsible for the weak impact of the program. Because of this mismatch, two lessons were clear. First, "challenging social problems cannot be best solved by narrowly focused 'crash' programs with large budgets." The report argued that "a greater impact on problems of distressed areas is likely to be made by a locally based, multipurpose institution—a community development corporation—than would result from government acting directly. Second, local institutions would need capacity-building development and strengthening."[14]

Over the past 40 years, the affordable housing sector has evolved significantly, and the lessons learned from the devastating impact of large-scale "towers in the park" upon urban cities across the country were broadly felt. But it was too late to undo the impact in East Harlem, where the highest concentration of low-income public housing in America is squeezed into 1.54 square miles.[15] My walk to work past them is a daily reminder of visionary excess, poor communication, and the seismic influence of the era's power brokers.

The Department of Housing and Urban Development, first established in 1965 and led then by Harold Freeman's cousin Robert Weaver, has continued to evolve over the years. In 1977 Congress passed the Community Reinvestment Act (CRA), and a national network of community development organizations sprang up across the country. The CRA is "intended to encourage depository institutions to help meet the credit needs of the communities in which they operate, including low- and moderate-income neighborhoods, consistent with safe and sound operations."[16] But limited interpretation and patchwork implementation of the CRA has left its effects mixed. Community development corporations (CDCs) and community development financing institutions (CDFIs), overseen by the Federal Reserve, have since used billions of tax-credit dollars to leverage private investments toward local development, particularly in neighborhoods like Harlem, where breaking cycles of disinvestment is crucial. In Harlem, for example, the Abyssinian Development Corporation (a CDC) led the development of the Pathmark grocery store, and based in Manhattan, the Nonprofit Finance Fund (a CDFI) makes investments and creates financing mechanisms to strengthen services and local organizations. Because of their sheer scale, it is not always easy to balance financial and corporate responsibilities with local needs. To do this, a range of intermediaries between community groups, CDCs, CDFIs, banks, and businesses have led the way in developing more locally tailored projects.[17] Eventually, the complex and evolving patchworks of tax credits and public subsidies have massively decentralized neighborhood development.[18]

As Harlem suffered at the hands of historic public housing development and a patchwork approach to social services, a growing supply of clinical care failed to stop the deterioration of individual health in the face of social change. Ray returned from Vietnam to a declining neighborhood, remained in low-income housing with few job prospects, grew sick as the nearby hospitals waited for him to arrive, all while the support groups he did interact with remained disconnected from the substantial resources around them. While other parts of Manhattan accelerated forward and began to accumulate wealth, Harlem's reputation lent itself to pity and contempt from outside, leading to a concentration of well-intentioned, poorly executed development projects. The same opportunities and protections that more wealthy neighborhoods were privy to never materialized. It is sadly not surprising that methadone clinics would concentrate in a neighborhood least equipped and resourced to handle the complex support its constituents really needed, while healthcare systems profited. Williams had a point.

POLITICS OF PROGRESS

One mechanism for building a healthier neighborhood in the face of these challenging forces is through politics—the art of achieving and leveraging power. Traditionally, the hallmark of such power has been the ability to divert resources into particular communities. But in Harlem, as in neighborhoods across the country, even significant political power and the resulting influx of resources has not been sufficient to improve health to the level enjoyed by wealthier parts of New York City.

Harlem's status as a major center of African American cultural and political activity contributed to its growing influence in the city, state, and nation over the twentieth century. Neighborhood-facing politicians, like Marcantonio, who carefully tended to their constituents and the city's idiosyncratic political dynamics, faded. In their place a new generation of African American politicians in Central Harlem found a national audience for their tempered political stance, in contrast to firebrands like Harlem's own Malcolm X.[19] When Ray was a young man, Charles Rangel, a Harlem-born Korean War veteran and attorney, was completing two terms in the New York State Assembly. Rangel defeated the charismatic 12-term congressman and pastor of the influential Abyssinian Baptist Church, Adam Clayton Powell Jr., to begin his first of nearly two dozen terms as Harlem's congressman. Rangel rose farther and more rapidly than any previous Harlem politician, joining a small fraternity of African American politicians in Congress. He joined the House Ways and Means Committee and by 1979 he was the Chair of the Subcommittee on Health. Once there, he began decades of support for Harlem Hospital, where Harold Freeman was developing his patient navigator program. He joined Republicans to overhaul the tax code in 1986, where he authored the Low-Income Housing Tax Credit, which the Federal Reserve scholar Erickson credits as a decentralizing force in the affordable housing industry.[20]

Life in Rangel's congressional district had deteriorated significantly since he was a young man. He frequently expressed his frustration over what he saw as the loss of individual responsibility, but he also knew that preaching alone would not suffice. Rangel's memorable style made him a media fixture. The *New York Times* reported, "He says Hispanic and black teenagers are alone among God's creatures in having no sense of self-preservation and he calls drug dealers so dumb they have to eat in Burger Kings because they can't read a menu."[21] He used his growing political power to launch national initiatives with an eye on the economic development of his own Harlem, which became the testing ground for a series of government antipoverty pilots and programs. Change was constant, but it was difficult to say what, if anything, was working. Rangel certainly held power—and could credibly claim to have the best interests of the neighborhood at heart—but could he understand what that system needed to achieve the purpose of healthier lives?

HEALTH AND ECONOMIC DEVELOPMENT

In *The American Healthcare Paradox*, Elizabeth Bradley and Lauren Taylor assert that compared to peer countries, the United States falls last in terms of social spending, while vastly overspending on medical care. "The crucial need for attention to broader determinants of health is well documented, but the funding shift required to implement such a vision remains elusive in a political landscape characterized by diffuse power." [22] Harlem, like most American neighborhoods, confronts us with a more complicated picture. Over the course of the last half-century, political power and influence deliberately shifted from East to Central Harlem, leaving a legacy of social and economic interventions that began with the expansion of public housing in East Harlem and more recently has been exemplified by the Upper Manhattan Empowerment Zone in Central Harlem. And yet, in 2015, the levels of poverty in East and Central Harlem were virtually identical. [23] In both East and Central Harlem, approximately a third of adults are obese, and diabetes rates (obesity is a risk factor) are similar. The same goes for strokes, where high blood pressure is a risk factor. Both neighborhoods have children and adults who suffer from asthma, which can progress to be life threatening without the right care. Avoidable hospitalizations due to asthma in children and adults ranked amongst the city's worst in both neighborhoods. More definitively, the rates of premature death compared to 59 other New York City neighborhoods are 54th and 52nd, respectively. Central Harlem appears to be doing slightly better than East Harlem in areas like self-reported well-being, but not by as much as the exuberant real estate market and signs of economic transformation would suggest.

A colleague of Bradley's at Yale, political scientist Jacob Hacker, presents a contrasting view of social spending in his book, *The Divided Welfare State: The Battle over Public and Private Social Benefits in the United States.* "Net public and private spending [on healthcare and social services], at 25.4 percent of GDP, is above the average for all eleven [peer] nations (24 percent). [24] His point is reinforced by Jacob Funk Kirkegaard, a scholar at the Peterson Institute for International Economics, who comes to a similar conclusion that America allocates more to social spending than generally acknowledged by incorporating the value of tax subsidies on private income, which are a major source of spending on healthcare and social services (and income tax subsidies disproportionately benefit the wealthy). [25] All of these scholars, however, come to the same conclusion: healthcare spending is both excessive and inefficient, and America is much less effective in improving health outcomes than its economic peers. It is clear that a neighborhood seen as a tangle of sector-based services, regardless of the source—government, nonprofit, or private sector—instead of a platform that serves the common good, leaves its residents to pay the price of closing the gap. Central problems remain: What constitutes beneficial local development? Can the neighbor-hood be a coherent platform for health improvement?

Over the decades, political powers have made attempts at creating some version of such a platform. Their success has been limited by narrow views of the key factors that create vitality in a neighborhood—often, local eco-nomic development is viewed as a platform on its own. In 1992, Rangel, along with his republican counterpart Jack Kemp, co-authored legislation creating Empowerment Zones, which ultimately led to the 1993 Community Renewal Initiative, administered by HUD. The legislation, supported by the Clinton administration, was predicated upon public financing attracting private investment into businesses and nonprofit organizations in rural and urban areas across the country. The Upper Manhattan Empowerment Zone Development Corporation (UMEZ) came into existence in 1995 and had invested $230 million in Upper Manhattan (Washington Heights, East Harlem, and Central Harlem) by 2012. The zone's center is at the heart of Rangel's voting constituency. Provisions included tax-exempt facility bonds, incentives for organizations that create employment in the zone, and an infusion of social service block grants—all aimed at pulling the resources needed to turn the neighborhood into a platform for growth.

The community participated heavily in efforts to coax investment into the neighborhood. C. Virginia Fields, Manhattan Borough president from 1997 to 2005, recalls, "We did drawings and we scheduled tours, in big Greyhound-type buses, where we brought developers up from downtown as if they were immigrants coming from a foreign land."[26] These days, partially subsidized real estate development is booming and property values are rising rapidly, likely driven by these investments. The upscale grocery store Whole Foods opened on Malcolm X Boulevard, for those who can afford it. The feeling of prosperity pulses through the streets as new restaurants and condominiums spring up, part of the wave that brought my family to the neighborhood. What remains unclear is how these new dollars will translate into improved health for *everyone* in the neighborhood five and ten years from now.

The basic logic of concentrated local development efforts is that neigh-borhoods attract business development and local employment is gener-ated. Health status and income are closely correlated, making a steady job crucial for composing a healthy life. However, there is little done to verify if this is more than ideology.[27] For example, job creation alone, particularly low-quality jobs with limited career ladders, is deceptive. The uplift of a community also requires taking on the power differentials that perpetuate structural disadvantages. As the methadone clinics in East Harlem demonstrate, the type of influence that other Manhattan neighborhoods and even next-door Central Harlem have attained remains elusive. These dynamics play out block-by-block: UMEZ projects like the East Harlem Pathmark grocery store pledged that 75 percent of their employees would come from within the neighborhood. However, having an entry-level job income does not alone create the conditions to survive and thrive in an otherwise poor neighborhood. Given the scale of development, an opportunity was lost to transform the area beyond the construction of a building.

Simply clearing the official poverty line does not translate into good health or real opportunity. What individuals and families need in order to be successful varies—the combination and timing of opportunities have to coincide with their readiness and capability to take advantage of them. When our democratic processes become ossified and feeble in the face of persistent social and economic disadvantage, Americans become more vulnerable. At the border of basic self-sufficiency, minor setbacks turn catastrophic, and poor health is a major cause and consequence of decline. In the end, local economic development alone is not a panacea for poor health.

AN INTEGRATED PLATFORM

While UMEZ was developing its approach, the Harlem Children's Zone (HCZ) was forming, led by Geoffrey Canada from 1990 until 2014. Canada was motivated to build a birth-to-college system for poor children who lived within what was originally a 24-block area of Central Harlem; it eventually expanded to 97 blocks. He gained national attention through strong media coverage of his efforts coupled with impressive outcomes for the program's students in both health and education. The zone has been a boon for many: what makes it different from previous attempts at development is its aim of transforming the scattered services of a neighborhood into a platform that is more than the sum of its parts. Whereas other programs have sought to add more pieces to the puzzle, HCZ has sought to provide the glue that binds those pieces together.

The HCZ is largely privately funded, receives intensive technical support, and is guided by a highly motivated and skilled leadership team. The success of their model in new settings will depend upon how effectively inexperienced neighborhoods with a fraction of HCZ's funding can learn from what HCZ has been able to accomplish. Meanwhile, most children in the United States, including Ray's surviving grandkids just a few blocks out of the HCZ, do not live in a zone where children's development is an explicit priority. Their neighborhoods—the resources and institutions they are able to bring together to support their lives—are very different from what kids have just a zipcode away. It's devastating to think that there are opportunities nearby that they will never see, just as Ray never benefited from Freeman's navigators in his lifetime.

During the 1990s, the nation learned to incorporate local needs into community development projects, like UMEZ, through the input of neighborhood boards, the identification of relevant tax credits, and independent efforts by responsible developers. Over the past decade, the community development industry has intensified focus on building sophisticated transactions with better data and explicit concern for investing in livelihoods (that is, education, job training, and health). As a result, the classic view of community development and urban reform, which has historically focused upon real estate development, now includes other functions that have wide local benefit, including many that have been integrated by efforts like the HCZ. These scattered but intense efforts have contributed to growing, albeit rudimentary, nationwide expertise on how to proactively build healthy and cohesive neighborhoods.[28]

Today, Harlem is also economically diverse, and wealthy families increasingly live alongside those who struggle financially. Ultimately, these disparities in wealth lead to vastly different neighborhood experiences for different individuals. Even two people who live next door to one another can have great gaps in the resources available to them to build a healthy life. Whereas wealthy families significantly profit from disproportionately beneficial income tax breaks that allow them to smooth over neighborhood deficits (below-average schools, for example), a family living at or around the poverty line must spend many hours if not days in a month trying to assemble a scatter of essential social benefits, while working one or more jobs to keep from teetering into destitution. As private, out-of-pocket expenditures rise for healthcare and self-care across the nation, illness—particularly a chronic condition like diabetes—is a substantial financial burden that regularly requires neighbors to choose between their personal health and their family's survival.[29] Although living on the same streets, these families do not experience the same neighborhood.

CHEAP TALK

In the absence of political or economic cure-alls, how might everybody's neighborhood be changed for the better? A few months after the fatal stabbing outside of the methadone clinic near Ray's home, Williams organized a meeting at his apartment to discuss what he called quality-of-life issues. There was a wide cross section of the neighborhood in attendance, including members of senior housing, long-time community advocates, Congressman Rangel himself, District Attorney Cy Vance Jr, a senior member of the NYPD, well-known ministers, and a handful of neighbors who brought friends, who in turn brought their friends. The informal nature of the gathering, coupled with the presence of influential local leaders, created a surprisingly vibrant and lively discussion. Arnie Segarra, a trusted leader of Casabe House and a self-described "neighborhood old-timer," spoke passionately about the safety concerns his peers expressed, always on their minds but heightened by the recent stabbing on their block. His comments about safety provoked others. People were angry about groups of young men on dirt bikes who ran through traffic lights at high speed, right in front of police: "Why don't you arrest them?" A memorable conversation ensued:

> *Neighbor [shouting]:* You're the cops, why can't you just arrest these kids on dirt bikes? They don't have licenses and they jump over car lanes and weave in between them. They're gonna kill people and you don't do anything about it!
>
> *NYPD official:* First of all, thank you for your comments. We have been tracking this issue, and it is difficult to always get there in time to do anything about it. If you provide me, personally, the information about when this happens [provides personal cell phone number], I'll let the local unit know to follow up.
>
> *Neighbor [shouting even more loudly]:* That's bullsh*t, I see your cops just watch them ride by, don't tell me you don't see them.
>
> *[NYPD official getting slightly agitated]*
>
> *District Attorney:* Sir, we take these complaints seriously. If a police unit just chases these kids, and one of them gets killed doing something stupid,

> then we have a serious problem on our hands. What we need is infor-
> mation about where they go, where they store their bikes; we need to
> address these issues in a safe way. I am sure someone knows where these
> boys live.

This exchange, just one month after the incendiary shooting of Michael Brown in Ferguson, Missouri, by police officer Darren Wilson, tapped into neighborhood tensions that go much deeper than traffic violations. They lead us right back to how resources are allocated and managed to improve life in our neighborhoods. It was an animated and far-reaching conversation, with issues ranging from the dirt bike gangs, to the unsafe area around the methadone clinics, to long-standing concerns about asthma in public housing that resurfaced with the rising dust from new developments of expensive condominiums nearby.

Most issues the group identified had clear impacts on health outcomes, even if the event's participants did not categorize them in the same way. But as a healthcare professional, I was not clear on how the health and safety of my neighbors as discussed in Williams's apartment connected with the health and safety of these individuals as patients in clinic settings. Community members are not asked to voice their opinions and concerns when it comes to the financing or governance of healthcare resources. Why not? What would happen if they were?

GIVING THE WORK BACK TO NEIGHBORHOODS

In the 1970s, just as crime was skyrocketing in Harlem, Elinor Ostrom, a political scientist by training, began her groundbreaking work on how people govern scarce resources. Ultimately she was awarded a Nobel Prize for Economics for this work and recognized as one of *Time* magazine's 100 most influential people in the world. She studied the reform and governance of police departments, among other systems, examining where the interactions and norms between people are most critical. What enabled the efficient and sustainable management of resources? Part of her answer turned out to be "cheap talk"[30]—direct, informal communication where there was no immediately contractual or enforceable obligation between parties.

Instead of creating simple rule-based policy for complex social problems, an approach that has been a dominant tradition among academics and policy makers, Ostrom advocated that policing should be done *with*, not *to*, a community. This required that control of a technical, professionalized resource be shared with the neighborhood in order to be effective, and the means put in place to make this possible. In the realm of law and order, particularly in black neighborhoods that experienced high levels of police brutality when the issue was studied in the 1970s, this was a remarkable finding. On the question of moving from a large centralized police department (that is, vertically integrated and controlled) to smaller, neighborhood-oriented precincts (that is, more horizontally spread) she had this to say:

> Not a *single* case was found where a large centralized police department
> outperformed smaller departments serving similar neighborhoods in
> regard to multiple indicators. . . . We found that while many police depart
> ments served the 80 metropolitan areas that we also studied, duplication
> of services [like radio communication or criminal laboratory analyses]
> by more than one department to the same set of citizens rarely occurred.
> . . . We demonstrated that complexity is not the same as chaos in regard to
> metropolitan governance."[31]

Ostrom's ideas were extended to a wide range of systems, including healthcare, by her colleague Michael McGinnis at Indiana University. These concepts have served as the basis for the concept of a "local integrator" organization that coordinates the governance and financing of health improvement activities at the neighborhood level. Thought leaders behind healthcare reform, like Elliott Fisher at the Dartmouth Institute, have championed their creation.[32] The basic idea would be that neighborhood-level governance would be able to contract for health improvement services, which would include clinical care when necessary, as well as a wider range of local priorities. This requires more than policy and savvier healthcare consumers—it requires a new emphasis on health challenges and opportunities locally, rather than at the state or national level.

Take, for instance, the Blue Zone Project, which worked backward to discover common features among communities where residents lived unusually long lives. Loma Linda, California, is one such community, and there are many more worldwide. What the researchers found was that blue zones encouraged constant moderate physical activity, social engagement, consumption of vegetables, avoidance of smoking, and, above all else, placed an emphasis on family.[33] A *consequence* of how blue zones self-organized was high-quality, long lives. Putting economic and political power in the hands of Americans to shape how they relate to their own context is an enduring national idea that the healthcare sector has strongly resisted. As a physician, I find it all too easy to convince myself that patients or their families do not value their health if they disagree with well-defined clinical goals. The nation's poor bang for the healthcare buck indicates that it is simply impractical to sustain the belief that entire neighborhoods do not care about their health or future. However, this belief endures among healthcare leaders and policy makers, as indicated by how we finance and intervene in neighborhoods.

As a physician, I struggle to understand Ray's context. As a member of his former neighborhood, I am less sure that my professional concerns are aligned with his surviving family. Their sense of purpose, avenues for participation, and perspective on what a healthier life means are vitally important, yet elusive from my professional vantage point. How can a healthcare system and its neighborhood interact in ways that satisfy both the former's need to achieve high-value health outcomes (quality diabetes care) and the latter's interest in a meaningfully healthier life (a safe and socially active neighborhood)? Some sort of systems architect is required, an integrator whose perspective can "move from a vague concept and limited resources to a satisfactory and feasible system concept and executable program."[34]

For the past century, this role has been claimed by the field of public health, albeit in many ways, often with overlapping and inconsistent aims.

4

Contexts of Consequence

I grew up in Harlem. My grandmother was one of the best cooks around, but the first thing she did on Sunday mornings when she started cooking a daylong meal was to take a big block of lard from the back of the refrigerator and throw it into the pan.
—Dr. Richard Carmona, Nurse, Paramedic, Physician, Surgeon, Vietnam Veteran, Police Officer, and Former Surgeon General of the United States

AN ARMY OF ONE

The skills Ray developed in military service did not seem to be valued at home. Whereas some of his fellow veterans had opportunities in downtown Manhattan, he was always directed back uptown or to the outer boroughs where he was told his own kind could help him. He was aware of some job training programs, but no jobs. Getting a college education was out of the question: he had a young wife, children, and mouths to feed. People around him knew that he was having a hard time, but so were they. His values stopped him from participating in paths to personal gain that he felt were unethical, and he was simply fortunate not to be incarcerated by association with friends who had committed minor, often drug-related, infractions.[1] At the same time the skills he did have were discounted at every turn.[2] His wife was able to get work in a downtown office, but they lost their meager savings in a fishy process to buy an apartment in Harlem that turned sour for reasons they never understood.[3] It seemed better to stay in low-income housing, despite its drawbacks. His own health was the last thing on his mind, and yet the conditions for poor health intensified. His life history and

69

the varied contexts he had lived through were water under the bridge when Ray finally got to the emergency department many years later.

As Harold Freeman attested decades ago, socioeconomic, behavioral, and physical environment factors deeply influence the health of people well before, during, and after periodic healthcare interactions. It is no surprise, then, that chronic medical conditions, which can include cancer, heart disease, addiction, depression, and diabetes, present a fundamental challenge to the American healthcare system. Today, seven out of ten deaths are due to chronic conditions.[4] In 2009, nearly half of all Americans had a chronic medical condition, which consumed nearly 85 percent of our healthcare budget.[5] In Harlem, smoking is still much more common than it is in the rest of New York City or the country[6]—and it is a major social driver of chronic disease and early death: one of many signs that the health of my neighbors will get worse before it can get better. For a range of reasons, the proportion of Americans with one or multiple chronic conditions is projected to increase.

This isn't, however, an iron law: as Thomas Farley, New York City Health Commissioner under Mayor Michael Bloomberg, stated, "It's not a given that we're going to continue to have high rates of smoking and high rates of [chronic] diseases; those are as preventable as infectious diseases were 150 years ago."[7] However, his optimism best reflects the trajectory of wealthier neighborhoods like the Upper East Side, which have experienced remarkable increases in lifespan and quality of life. To the north, neighborhoods like Harlem and the South Bronx lag far behind. Areas of upper Manhattan and the Bronx have barely recovered from HIV/AIDS and drug epidemics, as well as sky-high homicide rates,[8] all in the context of rapid urban upheaval, economic collapse, and hardball policing tactics that scar and reinjure the neighborhood's social fabric. The gaps between adjacent neighborhoods like the Upper East Side and East Harlem are widening, and like the difference in adult smoking rates, very low performance of public schools in the latter indicates that disparities in health outcomes are likely to grow, rather than recede, over the next generation.

What about the role of personal choice? Alvin Pouissant, an East Harlem–raised Harvard psychiatrist and co-author of *Come on People! On the Path from Victims to Victors* with Bill Cosby, has publicly shared his journey of attending Columbia University while living with his two brothers, Kenny and James, who were addicted to heroin. He earned a full scholarship to attend nearby

Weill Cornell Medical School.[9] However, as we celebrate Pouissant's ac-complishments, we must also recognize that his personal narrative, which included studying in the same apartment where his brothers succumbed to ravaging addiction, makes his story exceptional.

In 2010, Rutgers Professor of Human Ecology Naa Oyo Kwate worked with a young public health practitioner, Donya Williams, to show that there are more fast-food restaurants in predominantly black neighborhoods like Central Harlem than in other neighborhoods. A year earlier, Kwate had shown that 25 percent of all visual advertisements in Central Harlem mar-keted alcoholic beverages, with an even higher concentration near schools. Proximity to fast food and exposure to alcohol marketing, Kwate argued, drives increased consumption of each. Consequently, demand for alcohol and fast food within a neighborhood increases, attracting still more busi-nesses catering to these demands.

If Pouissant and Kwate sat down to review what we know about the fac-tors that led to Ray's death, they would probably disagree upon what should have been done differently while he was alive. In all likelihood Ray would have agreed with the views of Pouissant. Ray held a deep conviction that his health and his circumstance were his own responsibility, according to his daughter. He probably had little awareness or concern about how much the odds were tilted against him in insidious ways.

Ray started gaining weight a few years after coming back from Vietnam, which threw off his internal metabolic balance. Weight gain and loss is controlled by a combination of conscious and subconscious factors. Being depressed or stressed leads some people to gain weight while it leads others to lose weight rapidly. There are many reasons why Ray gained weight and gradually moved toward a path of multiple chronic conditions. Obviously no one sector—like healthcare—can take on something as complex as obesity alone, as Kwate's work supports. It is also fair to say that Ray played a central role in assembling the factors that would lead him to either a healthy or unhealthy life, as Pouissant's story suggests. The truth is that our healthy behavior is a function of motivation, influence, information, and a breadth of contextual factors—all working together.[10]

If I turned the tables and asked of myself, as a physician, what I'd expect if I met Ray as a young man, middle-aged father, or elderly gentleman, I know that the reasonable goals we would develop together to put him on a healthier path would be hard to achieve if he simply relied upon himself.

Contrary to nearly all clinical guidelines that view each patient as an army of one, most of my neighbors see their own health as intertwined with the health of people around them. Many are caregivers themselves. In the United States, more than 80 percent of the long-term care is provided by informal caregivers. It is no surprise that I meet neighbors and patients who fare poorly when the stress of self-care, caring for others, or consequences of avoiding healthcare become too much. This informal care is estimated to be worth $200 billion, at the real cost of pervasive burnout and stress.[11]

As our nerves fray, so does our willingness to be civically engaged citizens who are part of larger group efforts. According to Harvard political scientist Robert Putnam, joining and participating in one group cuts in half your odds of dying next year, and joining two groups cuts it by three-quarters.[12] It is again no surprise that after Ray's wife died, his health and well-being fell apart, as his only dedicated link to the diverse and overlapping social world of the neighborhood passed away with her. As Putnam emphatically conveys in *Better Together*, a rich and supportive social network is a vital ingredient for a healthy life:

> Again and again, we find that one key to creating social capital is to build in redundancy of contact. A single pitch is not enough, whether you are pitching unionization or Christian salvation. Common spaces for commonplace encounters are prerequisites for common conversations and common debate. Furthermore, networks that intersect and circles that overlap reinforce a sense of reciprocal obligation and extend the boundaries of empathy.[13]

Fortunately for Ray, he had committed family support: his children took on the parallel tasks of managing his affairs, including the complex details of his veteran and social benefits, and getting him to his prescribed clinic visits. But the work of caregiving can feel endless, and a family's patience and cohesion can unravel unexpectedly in the process, leaving everyone more vulnerable. These are just some ways that poor health in some impacts us all, yet again indicating that the scope of this challenge extends well beyond helping people navigate the healthcare system once they are sick.

Moreover, even the best aspects of clinical care have their limits. According to University of California, San Francisco, nephrologist Carmen Peralta, biomedical research circa 2015 was not able to effectively answer questions about the roots of kidney failure—one of the unaddressed mysteries of Ray's decline.[14] While we continue to invest in advances in clinical medicine and scientific discovery, we must also search outside the patient's body—to his family experience and neighborhood history—for forces that may already be shaping his grandchildren's future.[15]

The impact of how one American life unfolds can deepen across generations, just as advantage and disadvantage tend to have compounding effects. Whereas Ray was willingly drafted into the army to serve his country at a time of war, his grandchildren are part of a generation in which only 1 percent of Americans serve in our voluntary military, from a national pool where 75 percent are unfit to serve. Obesity is the leading reason.[16] While military service has historically been a path to social and economic opportunity, increasingly there will be an uphill struggle for eligibility. Our East Harlem neighborhood has the highest rate of diet-related diseases in New York City, making Ray's grandchildren unlikely to follow in his footsteps. At Ray's funeral, one of his grandsons proudly wore Ray's military decorations upon a chest that was alarmingly large for a preteen. It occurred to me that Ray had had opportunities that his grandchildren are unlikely to have. Taken together, growing health inequity across neighborhoods and across generations has a profoundly negative impact on the future of the country, striking at the heart of the source of our nation's dynamism: each other.

PUBLIC CONTEXTS, PUBLIC HEALTH

Public health professionals believe that it is possible to tilt a person's context toward or away from health, making it more or less likely for an individual to be healthy in the long run. This is an inclusive and general sentiment, as reflected in the Institute of Medicine's 1988 report on the future of public health, which defined public health as "what society does collectively to assure the conditions for people to be healthy."[17] Public health scholars and practitioners use their diverse backgrounds—community organizing and media advocacy, medicine and nursing, law and social sciences, economics and epidemiology, to name just some—to take a broad view of the landscape of factors that influence a population's health. When an opportunity to act emerges, an intervention, in the form of a targeted program or policy, is unleashed. As Columbia historian James Colgrove writes in *Epidemic City*: "These actors select from an array of potential policy approaches—the public health 'tool kit'—ranging from persuasive measures such as mass media education and social marketing to more coercive interventions such as quarantine or regulation of property or commerce. People involved in these processes take advantage of windows of opportunity, such as perceived state of epidemiological, fiscal or moral crisis, to advance a particular course of action."[18]

Public health's periscope has an ever-expanding field of view. Interdisciplinary teams of public health scientists, like Harvard's Ichiro Kawachi and Lisa Berkman, have used the "neighborhood" as a focused unit for integrating perspectives on health at the level of individual relationships, community-level interactions, and social and political action.[19] In this context, sociologists have shown us how a thicket of relationships influences opportunity, mobility, and life span.[20] Network scientists like Yale's Nicholas Christakis and his colleague at the University of California, James Fowler, have even suggested that *noncommunicable* chronic conditions can spread within a social network through a combination of cultural and behavioral factors. Harvard professors William Julius Wilson and Robert J. Sampson emphasize that simply being together or knowing a lot of people is less important than what can be accomplished together, which they call "collective efficacy."[21] Working in convergent directions, sociologists, economists, and political scientists have emphasized that *social capital* and the emergent property of *civic virtue* are the glue that hold society together, which in turn can influence health status.[22]

The breadth of what public health encompasses is astounding, and one quickly concludes that *everything* impacts health. Instead of thinking about the health of an individual, public health is concerned with the health of people in our many interconnected social, physical, spiritual, and economic contexts. It is plain to see that public health and healthcare are inextricably linked, but street-level practitioners have radically different perspectives informed by different day-to-day experiences.

Where and how should we meet?

AN INTERVENTION

Kwate's former student Donya Williams helped me understand the rapidly evolving and dynamic way that public health practitioners think of improving the health of the neighborhood. She had left the New York City Department of Health in December 2012 after running a street-level campaign to improve healthy food access in Harlem, and she knew the subject better than any of my hospital colleagues. I met her at Il Café Latte on Malcolm X Boulevard in the neighborhood. The coffee shop was busy, filled with Dutch tourists who had come to see the American version of their native Haarlem, drawn by travel guides that recount tales of its gospel music, soul food, and the history of the Harlem Renaissance.

Williams's family, like Ray's, had come to New York by way of North Carolina on a common migratory path of African Americans moving from the rural South to the industrial and urban North. This was only a couple generations after the robust slave trade that drove the development of New York City finally ended.[23] Her family settled in Newburgh, New York, and she eventually moved to New York City. As a child, she regularly attended funerals of fellow African American community members, which she described as "a very regular and normal part of life."[24] She was drawn to public health because she noticed that these individuals had often died prematurely, in spite of having a good education and job. Her own father died early from lung cancer. She recognized that his illness and treatment was about more than his medicines. "Even when he was sick, he did not know where things had gone wrong, and frankly, neither did we; that meant that there wasn't much wisdom about how to live better aside from whatever passed for commonsense." She joined the New York City Department of Health in 2007, before the ACA was passed, at a time of heightened enthusiasm for activist public health measures under the Bloomberg administration.

On the heels of the success of the citywide antitobacco campaigns, Mayor Bloomberg and the team of his health commissioner, Thomas Frieden, devised a suite of ads, programs, and legislative strategies to reduce obesity. Their success with tobacco echoed across the world, and it was clear that obesity was the next frontier. Ever since airplanes started charging obese passengers for two seats and Oprah started talking openly about her weight problems, Americans have been hearing about their expanding waistlines. In 2010, the Centers for Disease Control (CDC) estimated that one out of three Americans was obese,[25] and, collectively, obese Americans drove 10–20 percent of healthcare spending. Since being obese increases the risk of conditions like arthritis, heart disease, diabetes, and depression, preventing obesity presents a natural opportunity to shift the fulcrum to well-being and prevention rather than disease. Other cities and states emulated New York's program, including Arkansas under the leadership of Governor Mike

Huckabee. What made New York City's effort stand out, however, was its persistent use of regulatory tools and public health interventions to change the default food environment of city dwellers. In recognizing that marketers and ad agencies access our subconscious to influence our habits, the city utilized the same methods to promote a healthier message.

The Bloomberg administration's approach to tackling obesity included efforts to build a business ecosystem for healthy foods. This endeavor focused on the concept of food deserts—geographic areas with limited access to nutritious foods. Michelle Obama had pledged to eliminate food deserts as part of her Let's Move! campaign, bringing them to popular attention. The US Department of Agriculture mapped areas with low access to affordable, healthy food options and found that nearly one in ten Americans lived in such areas, including many in rural parts of the United States.[26] Not surprisingly, East Harlem is one of the worst food deserts in New York City, has the highest rate of diet-related diseases, and is considered to be a diabetes hotspot.[27] Ray and his neighbors grew up in this context. In contrast, Upper East Side residents thirty blocks south have endless choices of health-oriented services like specialty gyms and health food stores, which contribute to a virtuous cycle of well-being.

The Bloomberg administration felt that it could not stand by as some New Yorkers suffered. Neighborhood coalitions like Project HEED in East Harlem had clearly articulated the need for support. By the time Bloomberg took on New York's obesity crisis, he had in hand the data to make his case, evidence of local support to make it a political centerpiece, and the mayoral muscle to follow through. This was a classic case of data-driven, evidence-based policy making that put the health statistics of the public at the forefront. At first glance, the solution was simple: green the food deserts by increasing supply. The businessman-turned-mayor declared, "There is demand for fruits and vegetables in these neighborhoods, and this regulatory change will enable the market to meet that demand."[28]

The Bloomberg team chose to address food deserts through a fixture of New York neighborhoods: bodegas. If you're unfamiliar with the concept of a bodega, just imagine a mom-and-pop version of 7-Eleven, customized to the neighborhood's tastes. The word *bodega* is Spanish and derives from the same root as *apothecary*—pharmacist, but these stores provide a different kind of "fix." Bodegas are everywhere in New York. Some city surveys estimate that up to 80 percent of residents shop at their neighborhood stores.

The merchandise commonly available—products like cigarettes, honey buns, sodas, and beef jerky—reflects the impulse buys of many Americans. These items are prominently displayed in the store and at the checkout counter. What many bodegas *don't* sell are fruits and vegetables. To correct this, Bloomberg's administration launched a pair of complementary initiatives: the Green Cart program, aimed at building an army of fruit and vegetable street vendors, and the Healthy Bodega Initiative, that would transform the stores themselves. These programs, like calorie labeling, reflected a growing emphasis on "nudging" people toward better choices by offering healthier defaults options. Ultimately, they would prove to be an example of how well-intended, well-researched public health interventions fail when they do not include the street-level perspective in the design process.

Donya Williams was in charge of getting the Healthy Bodega Initiative off the ground in East and Central Harlem (it also operated in Central Brooklyn and the South Bronx). Like a theater crew trying to build a new set from old parts, Williams's team set out to make nutritious options appear to be the new default:

> My staff had to go store to store to convince bodega owners to rearrange their shelves to promote healthier items. At first, they looked at us like we were crazy, because we were essentially asking them to hide their best sellers in favor of potential duds or perishables that would go to waste and rot. We chatted, developed a relationship, and they slowly let me move a couple things up front or to better view than alternatives. You can't explain [to bodega owners] that their offerings are a gateway to obesity and diabetes; these are small business owners who have to understand how "healthy choices" don't hurt their livelihoods. It's a conversation that only a strong relationship allows.

Bodega owners have real experience with their customers' habits, and most of the owners that Williams interviewed reflexively believed that a guy like Ray would sail by "healthy" changes and stick with what he was accustomed to eating. If you're on a mission for Doritos or don't have the money to risk trying something new, the subtle "fresh" choices are easy to pass over. For the generation that included Ray's grandchildren, however, there was hope that having the opportunity to see better choices from a young age would subtly shape eating preferences.[29] Healthy Bodega provides advertising and supply-chain relationships for more nutritious food options, and Williams played a crucial role in building a ground operation that reaches about 1,000 bodega owners. This inroading is no small feat given that most are independent small businesses with deep roots in the neighborhood. But in terms of health outcomes, the immediate impact of these interventions has been disappointing. A study of a similar effort in Philadelphia by a team of environmental health and sociology researchers stated:

> We found that the intervention moderately improved residents' perceptions of food accessibility. However, it did not lead to changes in reported fruit and vegetable intake or body mass index … The present findings suggest that simply improving a community's retail food infrastructure may not produce desired changes in food purchasing and consumption patterns. Complementary policy changes and interventions may be needed to help consumers bridge the gap between perception and action.[30]

After being on the frontlines of the Healthy Bodegas Initiative, Williams held a similar view about the success of this approach:

> We were able to make some subtle but substantial changes in stores and the streets. There were definitely more healthy foods available, and more channels to get them at a reasonable price. But I get it, after a day in a stressful or tough environment, it's not about nutrition—it's about comfort and culture. That's much harder to address. It requires that the same deep conversations that I had with the bodegas happen in the household and across the neighborhood. And it was hard to see how the public health community was going to do that directly without barging into people's lives.

A Mount Sinai research group, the same that helped to organize Project HEED, found that Bloomberg's complementary city initiative to deploy mobile fruit and vegetable vendors didn't often manifest in the food deserts it was intended to reach.[31] Unsurprisingly, mobile vendors clustered near healthy stores and subway stops, hoping to capture customers who were already looking for fruits and vegetables, rather than converting those who were not. The pent-up "demand" that Bloomberg referenced was not so simple to unleash with a few well-aimed interventions.

The classic methods of public health interventions, epitomized by the Bloomberg initiatives, fell short of their potential because they aimed to protect people from external forces, as if neighbors were not agents in their own consumption. There's an undeniable logic to this approach: if public health doesn't directly influence an individual's behavior, someone else will. In 2012, when Bloomberg pushed for a portion cap on the size of soft drinks, I remember seeing Pepsi vans flood the city neighborhoods with sky-high childhood obesity rates. Millions of marketing dollars were spent on shaping public opinion with ads equating soda with freedom of choice. Public support for the anti-obesity initiatives waned. Popular media echoed the claim that the New York Health Department's suite of efforts amounted to a "nanny state," and the backlash echoed across the country as states like Mississippi preemptively banned similar public health measures. Tom Frieden, who would go on to lead the CDC, believed that the odds were stacked against New Yorkers at a level that most individuals could not see, understand, or act upon even if they did. So did his successor, Thomas Farley. Both public health leaders focused upon highly leveraged interventions, which require little effort from people who are already stretched thin. In their view, long-term behavior change is important, but hard to achieve systemically without first shaping the context.

They were acting in the same public health tradition that has removed asbestos from workplaces, eliminated lead in paint, imposed smoking bans in public places, and regulated lethal allergens in the peanut industry. Nearly all policies were born in controversy, forged through evidence and outcry. Public health officials have the lateral vision to see in aggregate what individually focused systems that influence health (healthcare, education, housing) do not. They have often prioritized the right answer, the long-term goal, ahead of the right process necessary to mobilize broad-based infra-structure and public support to achieve it. As a consequence, complex public health efforts, like the diverse array of anti-obesity interventions described above, often lose their coherence when challenged. Studies and statistics may reflect the success of specific interventions, but as Donya Williams lamented about her family's understanding about her own father's death, families are often left none the wiser for them.

As I learned at Ray's funeral and as Williams found through her work on the streets and stores of Harlem, the false divide between individual health and collective well-being forms the gap where groups of individuals are left stranded at particularly vulnerable times of life. Meanwhile a very real divide between healthcare and public health has persisted. The gears of healthcare reform were just beginning to turn when Williams and I met in 2011. As healthcare systems across the nation started making limited excursions into their surrounding neighborhoods, they largely ignored the architecture of interventions that public health organizations had developed over the preceding decades. In turn, both healthcare systems and public health regularly ignore complementary community development efforts.

HOW PUBLIC HEALTH EVOLVES

In 1965, two years before Ray was deployed to Vietnam and the same year that Medicaid and Medicare were enacted, John Lindsay became New York City's 103rd mayor. He served until 1973, a few years after Ray returned to East Harlem from his military duty. His political profile was similar to Bloomberg's, "a charismatic liberal Republican and rising star on the national political scene."[32] He, too, took a muscular approach to managing the health of the city. As part of a larger effort to consolidate a sprawling city bureaucracy, he created 10 "superagencies." One of these, the Health Services Administration (HSA), explicitly combined public health (preventive) and healthcare (curative) services to reduce waste and logically link two parts of population health improvement. He had the backing of many New York City public health officials, who would retain their identity within HSA: "Health prevention and promotion on the one hand and diagnostic and curative services on the other, must be brought together into a more comprehensive non-fragmented, easily available package for the consuming public."

Tension among leaders within the Department of Health grew, as those with the professional credentials and administrative skills appeared to have a leg up over equally committed colleagues. At this decisive moment, where the identity of public health was being actively contested, George James, the department's commissioner when Lindsay was elected, resigned to lead the Mount Sinai School of Medicine, a move that would presage the exodus of public health–oriented physicians to jobs at better-paying healthcare institutions. Howard J. Brown took over as the head of the newly formed HSA and laid down its priorities: "rebuilding deteriorating hospitals and financing and organizing medical care for 'ghetto areas.'" He came down decisively in favor of a healthcare-centric view of public health: "The public health leaders of the future," Brown predicted, would be "board certified public health physicians with training and skills in community medicine— medical sociologists, health urbanists—whatever they might be called . . . with one foot in the technical field of the science of medicine and the other in community dynamics." However, most of the department's committed public health practitioners did not fit his description, sowing resentment among its ranks.

His vision plunged the department into conflict, contributing to an en- during rift between "real" public health professionals, who took an expan- sive view of their field, and clinicians who saw public health as an adjunct to healthcare systems. The startlingly rapid growth of healthcare delivery for what was known as "ghetto medicine," driven by New York State's broad and expensive Medicaid program, codified the dissonance. The publically funded "ghetto medicine" program became so large that New York State alone ac- counted for one-fifth of the nation's expenditure and covered 30 percent of New York City's population. The state legislature intervened and removed 1.8 million people—more than half of those covered—from the Medicaid rolls, which led private hospitals to lobby Governor Nelson Rockefeller to protect them from shortfalls from "uncompensated care." Money for HSA to build its own healthcare facilities was diverted to private hospitals in exchange for regulatory oversight of hospital- or clinic-based care delivery. As HSA was stripped of resources, it turned to policy change, regulation, and targeted interventions. Hospital physicians protested the department's regulatory oversight, and the Department of Health within HSA developed an increas- ingly punitive relationship with healthcare as it went after derelict and fraudulent medical providers. The idea of coordinated planning between hospital-provided services and public health interventions to benefit the same people became the exception, not the rule.

In an era of civil rights mobilization and resistance movements, the health consequences of deteriorating neighborhoods like East Harlem came to a boil as white public health professionals tried to intervene in the lives of African American and Puerto Rican residents of the neighborhood. In 1969, an East Harlem group called the Young Lords mobilized after the city recorded high rates of lead poisoning in their neighborhood. They de- manded to oversee the health of their own neighborhood, in the form of a 10-point health plan (see box 4.1). The methods of social organization and the politics of social justice clashed with the technical perspective of

BOX 4.1

Ten-Point Health Plan for East Harlem
Created by the Young Lords, 1969

1. We want total self-determination of all health services in East Harlem (El Barrio) through an incorporated Community-Staff Governing Board for Metropolitan Hospital. (Staff is anyone and everyone working at Metropolitan.)

2. We want immediate replacement of all Lindsay administrators by community and staff appointed people whose practice has demonstrated their commitment to serve our poor community.

3. We demand immediate end to construction of the new emergency room until the Metropolitan Hospital Community-Staff Governing Board inspects and approves them or authorizes new plans.

4. We want employment for our people. All jobs filled in El Barrio must be filled by residents first, using on-the-job training and other educational opportunities as bases for service and promotion.

5. We want free publicly supported health care for treatment and prevention. We want an end to all fees.

6. We want total decentralization—block health officers responsible to the community-staff board should be instituted.

7. We want "door-to-door" preventive health services emphasizing environment and sanitation control, nutrition, drug addiction, maternal and child care, and senior citizen's services.

8. We want education programs for all the people to expose health problems—sanitation, rats, poor housing, malnutrition, police brutality, pollution, and other forms of oppression.

9. We want total control by the Metropolitan hospital community-staff governing board of the budget allocations, medical policy along the above points, hiring, firing, and salaries of employees, construction and health code enforcement.

10. Any community, union, or workers organization must support all the points of this program and work and fight for that or be shown as what they are—enemies of the poor people of East Harlem.

Ten-Point Health Program of the Young Lords, webpage, accessed December 15, 2015, http://www2.iath.virginia.edu/sixties/HTML_docs/Resources/Primary/Manifestos/Young _Lords_health.html.

public health officials, just as money for "ghetto medicine" was diverted to private hospitals like Mount Sinai. Only a few years later, in 1975, New York City's economy collapsed, leaving the Harlem neighborhoods in a free fall that ultimately led Harold Freeman and his colleague Colin McCord to ascribe "natural disaster" status to the excessive mortality rates in the neighborhood in 1990.[33] By that time, the intertwined HIV/AIDS, IV drug, and crime epidemics had taken a considerable toll on Harlem. Without deep ties to Harlem communities, neither inert local healthcare institutions nor a patchwork of meagerly funded public health programs nor disparate health activist groups like Young Lords could stabilize the increasingly stressful and dangerous neighborhood where Ray and his wife were raising their children.

By the time Bloomberg took office in 2002, the Harlem neighborhoods were coming out of a deep state of decline and despondence. Indeed, the health statistics he inherited were shocking, and he hired the brilliant Frieden as health commissioner, fresh from time in India where he had led a successful tuberculosis program as a medical officer for the World Health Organization. In many ways, Frieden represented the ideal public health professional that Howard J. Brown had envisioned for the HSA decades earlier. However, Frieden and his successors had both feet rooted in the technical field of the science of medicine and public health, rather than one in the former and the other in "community dynamics." Both Frieden and the socially minded doctors in New York City's healthcare systems saw the neighborhood and its people as requiring interventions to keep themselves healthy. Indeed, reductions in mortality are substantial for conditions that have been targeted simultaneously by the city's public health and healthcare systems—strokes and heart attacks especially. However, without an organizational or historical record of how these two groups worked together, it is difficult to identify where and why their initiatives worked, and where and why their initiatives fell short when the health of the neighborhood and the individuals within it, like Ray, deteriorated despite technically correct interventions.

Well chastened by the conflicts of the 1960s and 1970s, public health professionals continue to search for the right blend of data-driven decision-making and processes that can genuinely gain strength and support from the community. As healthcare systems like Mount Sinai rediscover their surrounding neighborhoods under the aegis of population health, their narrower clinical focus and stronger systems infrastructure may protect them from the type of backlash that public health professionals have faced in the past. However, these same protective qualities could easily result in an underwhelming and overpriced set of services that fail to take hold in the neighborhood. Still missing from both the public health and the clinical healthcare sectors is an official desire to harness community dynamics in a collaborative arrangement in which experts and community members co-design a neighborhood-centric, total population health system.

As I sat with Donya Williams to learn about her experience, I saw that our interest in the neighborhood united our perspectives even though we lacked the same training, experiences, or principles of engagement. As we spoke, we could both recognize the power that came from focusing on a common place rather than our different professional backgrounds. With our eyes trained on Harlem, it became obvious that we were no longer staring across a historic public health–healthcare divide; instead, we were natural allies in the health improvement of the neighborhoods where we lived.

TOWARD TOTAL POPULATION HEALTH

There are two classic ways of thinking about improving a neighborhood: one can view it as a place with *deficits* that need to be reduced, or one can see it as a place with *assets* that are pillars of investment. The former view dominates the clinical landscape, as disease burdens and disparities across the neighborhood are clear ways to describe problems in search of solutions. The most common assumption is that the solutions reside outside of the place where deficits exist, such as access to services, investment, or skills. Figuring out the most efficient way to provide them becomes a central concern. The latter view sees the neighborhood as a place where capabilities, assets, and skills are in various states of development that need to be nurtured. These include the power of relationships as a means to organize people and build upon what they have. In some ways, the former sees the neighborhood as a half-empty view and the other as half full. More importantly, they come with deep assumptions about how to motivate people, what kind of information and data lead to transformative change, and whether the past experience of the neighborhood matters. If we think about the neighborhood as a street-level platform of health improvement that is simultaneously working to reduce deficits and build upon its assets, it is crucial to understand who and what comprise the neighborhood platform, and identify methods that effectively inform and influence decision-making. For healthcare, public health, and the neighborhood to work together toward health improvement, they will require a common language through which to describe and understand their common goal.

At the same time, it is necessary to acknowledge that both healthcare and public health professionals are at least one step removed from the primary relationships between neighbors, family members, friends, acquaintances: those who comprise our public presence and private lives. If the neighborhood were merely a place to apply and clarify existing clinical protocols—taking better care of Ray's diabetes in his home setting, for instance —it would fit easily into the existing architecture of the healthcare sector in the form of *population medicine*. Supporting the *health* of a particular community where they live—elderly adults or vulnerable children, say—constitutes a *population health* that focuses upon subgroups, potentially spread over a region. However, if the goal is for *everyone* within a geographic area (such as a neighborhood) to live a healthier life, *total population health* must encompass how individuals and communities interact, how resources are governed and allocated, and what assets can be shared, by and for whom.[34] This is our aim.

Healthcare systems have much to gain from an interdependent relationship with strong public health systems. Most healthcare systems are too absorbed with their own internal challenges to invest in understanding the complex factors that lead to healthier lives in the neighborhood. To illuminate these blind spots, healthcare systems need the vision and guidance of strong public health systems that are anchored in the neighborhood. An effective public health system can "see" the neighborhood through multi-sector perspectives, analyze and connect seemingly unrelated components, and make the case for linkages that could improve the health of its many populations.

When successfully combined, a strong public health and healthcare system complement each other's blind spots, as argued by Morehouse School of Medicine Professor George Rust and former Surgeon General David Satcher and colleagues in "Triangulating on Success: Innovation, Public Health, Medical Care, and Cause-Specific US Mortality Rates over a Half Century (1950–2000)."[35] Their composite effect could be even more powerful if their capabilities were integrated within the same place. As demonstrated by the work of pioneers throughout this book, the successful interconnection of healthcare systems, public health, and neighborhood platforms to produce a coherent system of total population health will require forging new relationships between existing systems.

So, how can a neighborhood take a lead role in designing a total population health system? My neighbors have ideas for what would help them improve their own health and how to do it. What they don't always have, however, are the skills and scaffolds to act upon their intuition and ideas. The importance of embracing members of neighborhoods as co-creators of our healthcare systems, and the models for doing so, stands at the heart of the efforts I explore throughout this book. However, it is all too easy to advocate for oneself or one group at the expense of another, whether these tradeoffs are visible or not. Therefore, in order for members of a neighborhood to have an influential voice in co-creating total population systems—as healthcare consumers increasingly do today for healthcare systems—there must be increasingly tight feedback loops between their actions and the gradually improving performance of a total population health system over its composite parts.

Santa Fe Institute economist W. Brian Arthur observes that as a general rule, systems develop in this manner: "what starts as a series of parts loosely strung together, if used heavily enough, congeals into a self-contained unit."[36] In a total population health system, people should be able to assemble healthier lives more easily than they can today. As I followed Ray's memory through Harlem, I developed a loose sense of the types of interactions that are necessary to bring together healthcare systems, public health, and the neighborhood's development. I noted at least four such interactions:

1. *solving problems adaptively*: the extraordinary energy that drives innovation, discovery, and clinical improvement in healthcare needs to meet its match in the rich ways that communities organize to solve complex social and political challenges in the neighborhood;
2. *confronting tensions*: there needs to be much more "cheap talk," or channels of substantive communication between the neighborhood and local health systems, which is a vexing challenge, given that the neighborhood has myriad communities, aims, and priorities, and the healthcare and public health systems have a range of interfaces and goals;

3. *assembling health in place*: neighbors, local organizations, public health workers, and healthcare professionals need to co-create scaffolds of support for healthier lives in ways that honor their respective aims; and

4. *shifting the center of healthcare*: some activities that currently take place in the hospital should take place in the neighborhood, which requires a focus on quality and a major redesign in the relationships between healthcare professionals and a broader array of individuals and professions with the potential to improve population health.

Taking a step back from the impetus that Ray provided to explore our Harlem neighborhood up close, I wondered about how these interactions were playing out in other places across the country. I had also been hearing about pioneers across the country who have been immersed in building these interconnected parts of the neighborhood-based, total population health platform.

I had to see for myself.

PART II

5

The Value of Being Connected

*We have become technical experts on transactions when we need to lead
a new way of adaptive problem-solving.*
—Ben Hecht, "From Community to Prosperity"

Within New York City, Harlem has a unique healthcare and neighborhood
history. If you zoom out, New York City conducts itself as a special (and often
contentious) part of the state of New York, probably because of its multiple
roles as a regional hub, national landmark, and a global city. To understand
if the neighborhood interactions I had identified in Harlem were useful for
redesigning healthcare systems elsewhere, I sought to study settings across
America that felt sufficiently different from New York City in terms of: (1)
solving problems adaptively, (2) confronting tensions, (3) assembling health
in place, and (4) shifting the center of healthcare. Each of the chapters in
part 2 explores one of these interactions, in sequence, even as they overlap
considerably.

As I traveled across the country to places in each of the four statistical
regions and nine divisions that the US Census Bureau uses to subdivide the
nation, two encounters stood out—one in Texas and another in Minnesota.
In turn, these encounters led me to reflect upon the larger context that
surrounded the neighborhood work my colleagues and I were actively engaged in, and how insights from more advanced healthcare reform efforts
in Massachusetts, which served as the testing ground for the ACA, might
smooth our way forward.

It was in Dallas, Texas, that I encountered the work of Ruben Amarasingham and his colleague Anand Shah, who have taken a disciplined approach

to solving problems adaptively. In turn they discover opportunities for their healthcare systems to better support the surrounding neighborhoods. Their deep understanding of healthcare's technology and financial systems led them to an unexpected focus on connecting hundreds of Dallas-area organizations, a complex technical and collective action challenge. Their work took place in the context of persistent ethical leadership at Parkland Memorial Hospital, and amid growing national awareness that the business of healthcare must be realigned with its social mission. Amarasingham led the endeavor and aligned himself with a network of problem solvers determined to place challenging financial questions, persistent social challenges, and competing and contradictory healthcare system and neighborhood aims all into the same frame. Although the state-level healthcare reform environment in Texas is significantly different from the one in New York, I recognized that many street-level challenges that neighbors face are, remarkably, the same.

THE VALUE PROPOSITION

The success story of Amarasingham and Shah's efforts begins with a study of contrasts: Louisiana and Texas, two states overseen, at the time, by politically like-minded governors whose similar views on healthcare have played out in very different ways. The man they have in common is a Louisiana State University–trained physician named Fred Cerise. A bright spot in a public health and hospital system left devastated by Hurricane Katrina, Cerise was also a thorn in the side of the ambitious governor Bobby Jindal. Jindal wanted to bring the public hospital system, which was under LSU's oversight, under private management. This would be like bypassing the compromise New York City public hospitals had to make under financial duress, to become the quasi-public HHC, and instead turn over the entire public safety-net system directly to the for-profit HCA conglomerate. In his role as head of the state health department, there wasn't a lot Cerise could do to stop the executive office in its privatization plans. So in vocal opposition to the governor, Cerise publicly advocated for the ACA-subsidized Medicaid expansion for Louisiana's uninsured:

> By refusing to participate in the Affordable Care Act, Jindal will deny access to 456,000 low income individuals through the Medicaid expansion.

A recent analysis by the Kaiser Family Foundation put the 10 year cost at less than $1 billion for Louisiana. In fact, when that expense is offset against additional savings on state funds currently spent on the uninsured, it is probable that there would be a net financial benefit to the state. . . . However, instead of providing desperately needed leadership and clarity for his constituents, Bobby Jindal continues to confuse us.[1]

From the megaphone of editorial opinion pages, Cerise's advocacy put him on shaky footing with Jindal, who was vehemently opposed to implementing the ACA, calling it a "blow to our freedoms."[2] "By expanding President Obama's healthcare law, 41 percent of Louisiana's population would be dumped into Medicaid. Soon there will be more people riding in the cart than people pulling the cart. The President is gradually turning the world's greatest health care system into the world's largest welfare system. The left has been very clear—their end goal here is to make all healthcare in America government health care."[3]

Jindal sent Cerise packing.

Since the universe of healthcare professionals with substantial executive experience and a focus on public service isn't so large, Cerise did not stay a free agent for long. Louisiana's loss was Texas's gain, as Parkland Health and Hospital System in Dallas, one of the nation's largest public health systems, appointed him as their new CEO in 2014. Parkland is a historic hospital, known mostly as the place where former President John F. Kennedy died after being shot by Lee Harvey Oswald in 1963. It also serves as the primary teaching hospital for UT Southwestern, a flagship Texas medical school. It has a similar arrangement to New York City's historic Bellevue Hospital, one of the main Health and Hospital Corporation (HHC) hospitals, which is affiliated with NYU School of Medicine.

Like many large safety-net systems, Parkland was plagued by its sluggish response to safety and quality issues that were magnified by national improvement campaigns in the first decade of the new century. The Parkland system had been without a CEO since Ron Anderson, widely admired for his dedication to the social mission of the hospital, had stepped down in 2012. Throughout his 30-year tenure, Anderson had taken a principled stance against "patient dumping," a practice of transferring unstable, poor patients from private hospitals to facilities like Parkland, and he had even endured death threats for his stand. His devotion to Texas and his hardscrabble

Oklahoma upbringing were legendary, making Parkland's social mission a point of regional and state pride.

Despite Texas governor Rick Perry's position against ACA expansion—one that mirrored Jindal's—privatization of the state's safety-net system has fortunately stayed off the agenda. Instead, there have been notable efforts in several Texas cities to drive public-sector innovation in healthcare design, such as a voluntary increase in taxes by the citizens of Travis County to contribute to UT Austin's new Dell Medical School, which will focus on innovation in neighborhood-level healthcare. The fact is, healthcare innovation in Texas has the space and support to actively address challenging health and social issues, in contrast to the situation in Louisiana under Jindal. As a result, Texas attracts and consistently retains mission-driven healthcare leaders. The timing of Cerise's appointment, in early 2014, couldn't have been better for an intense group of elite mathematicians and computer programmers who were led by the lanky Amarasingham.

Amarasingham, built like a college basketball player, conveys the gentle welcome of a caregiver. He uses his expressive hands to break down big questions into little bits, punctuated by halting pauses that trade speed for precision. During his internal medicine residency at UT Southwestern between 1999 and 2002, he gained the enthusiastic support of Anderson to create a database of the health challenges of homeless Parkland patients. Neither he nor Anderson could predict that their shared social interest would form the heart of the business case for health reform over a decade later.

After finishing residency, Amarasingham left Texas to pursue a fellowship at Johns Hopkins, where he explored predictive analytics and studied business management, well before healthcare policy makers shifted billions of economic recovery dollars to ignite the electronic health record (EHR) market in 2009.[4] Despite an early interest in computer programming and business, which included a small software company that he started with his brother in high school (all the signs of someone a venture capital firm would readily invest in), he chose to return to Parkland in 2007 instead of entering the burgeoning health tech market. His champion in residency, Anderson, had invited him back to apply what he had learned to the 1 million patients that Parkland cared for out of the 2.3 million people in Dallas County. Over the next seven years, he revolutionized the technology of Parkland's information and decision-making systems, introduced predictive algorithms to direct patient care, and brought previously unconnected organizations into contact with each other. Overseeing a team that could go toe to toe with any Silicon Valley company,[5] he and his colleagues redefined what a healthcare system could do to stabilize a patient's return to his or her neighborhood.

By the time Cerise arrived in 2014, Amarasingham's team had designed a number of cutting-edge platforms that improved decision-making in a public hospital system notoriously devoid of reliable or automated information sharing. With practical achievements under the team's belt, and growing national recognition, they wanted to build an ambitious network that connected local organizations to Parkland's information and payment systems, so the work of making Dallas healthier could be shared across its neighborhoods. From 2007 to the present, Amarasingham's work has focused on building a multidisciplinary team whose members share a common aim.

Recruiting top tech talent to a public hospital system sounds like a Sisyphean task. It lacks the promise of stock options and big bonuses. Taking a different tack, Amarasingham's value proposition was simple, and it comes in the form of a story.

PIECES OF PATIENT DELTA

John Delta (or Doe) is one of the names assigned to people who show up in an emergency room without identification, usually unconscious or too confused to give a name. The identity of most of us would be clarified by a quick peek at a wallet or cell phone—verifying the existence of a bank account, a stable place to sleep at night, or at least a friend who could help. On a bad night, clinicians sometimes see numerous John Deltas or Jane Deltas flash up on the EHR that serves as a command center, workflow tracker, and patient safety reminder. Amarasingham met this particular John Delta in 2008, after he was admitted to the hospital in a cold and unconscious state. Almost nothing was known about who he was, but after some testing, it became rapidly clear that he was in a clinical crisis called myxedema coma. This occurs in a small number of people who have dysfunctional thyroid glands, usually with something else like an infection superimposed. The treatment includes synthetic thyroid hormone, which millions of Americans take regularly to keep their levels in check, costing about a dollar a day. It turns out he had been admitted to the hospital six times previously with the same problem. From a narrow clinical perspective, the diagnosis, treatment, and management of Delta's immediate condition were straightforward. The hospital got his condition under control, and then he was discharged. Inevitably, he was back as his health continued to deteriorate, only briefly propped up by short-term medical treatment. Delta faced what Amarasingham calls the "chronic daily disaster" of figuring out what to do about a condition he understood poorly, moving between local organizations and services that had no idea why he regularly fell apart. After being taken care of, the cycle would simply repeat.

Amarasingham saw that there was something about the design of our healthcare system that actually created and aided this negative loop. Maybe it was his undergraduate training in neuroscience combined with his clinical intuition as a physician, or perhaps it was his programming background augmented by an interest in predictive algorithms—whatever the antecedents, his encounter with Delta crystallized the systemwide root of the problem. In residency Amarasingham had co-authored a paper entitled "Disease Conditions Most Frequently Evaluated among the Homeless in Dallas," and he had a deeper understanding of the world outside of the hospital than most clinicians.[6] Still, it took time for Amarasingham's team to piece together that John Delta was bouncing across a range of local organizations, including the Salvation Army shelter right across the street from Parkland Hospital. The staff there were overjoyed to hear from Amarasingham, not to mention relieved that Delta needed a relatively cheap medication to stabilize his health; with that piece of information in place, they could focus on everything else.

Why did it take so much effort for everyone who regularly interacted with Delta to be on the same page? Even more striking, how was it that Parkland—like healthcare systems across the country—had almost no ability to predict who was likely to wind up caught in this loop in the first place, despite taking care of a million people in Dallas County? Although the speed and circumstances may differ, this loop unfolds in numerous scenarios daily: in a wealthy Fort Worth businessman who tips over into florid heart failure a day after eating a large steak meal, or a Galveston-based policewoman who develops diabetes after years of eating an unhealthy diet while working nights, or in this case, in a homeless man in Dallas, who showed up in the emergency room multiple times a year. No matter the background, when practical information about a patient is stuck in discrete compartments—in an EHR, with a family member, in the notes of a scatter of local organizations—the time between being in and out of the hospital shrinks as individuals become dependent upon healthcare, or until their bodies can't take it anymore.

Determined to resolve the fundamental healthcare flaws exposed by Delta, Amarasingham oversaw the development of software that would bring together clinical data from various departments along with other social, economic, and demographic information to help refine its accuracy. His team did more than simply create an algorithm that replaces how healthcare teams make decisions (which itself carries enormous ethical implications[7]). In addition they built a system that pushes timely insights—for a patient about to be discharged without prescription drug coverage, a stable place to live, or caregiver support—so that a care team can break the downward spiral of healthcare dependence. Their innovative technology, eventually called Pieces, was tested in 2009 within the Parkland system the same year Congress poured billions of dollars into an initiative to digitize the antiquated system of health records—an act that would spur a debate about privacy, information sharing, and propriety that still roils today. Although Pieces was developed with homeless patients like Delta in mind, it enabled clinicians to see that even patients who had homes faced significant challenges when they left the hospital.

MAKING THE CASE

The HITECH legislation, which was passed as part of the American Recovery and Reinvestment Act of 2009, is often credited with making healthcare reform possible. The goal was simple: digitize the system of paper charts that physicians use to keep track of patients and bring the healthcare sector into the twenty-first century. Following the infusion of more than $30 billion into the nascent EHR market, there ensued a frenzy of competition as companies built, acquired, collapsed, and endured until the basic architecture of the EHR market more or less stabilized with enterprise-level software like Epic Systems and Clarity, which now form the bulk of Parkland's system as well as Mount Sinai's. Whatever the flaws of the current generation of EHRs—that they detract from the patient care experience as doctors click their way through interviews, that information appears to go in without coming out, that they pose barriers to interoperability of information exchange between healthcare systems—it is impossible to overstate its historic importance for healthcare.

For Amarasingham's team at Parkland, the HITECH Act was a major boon to the Pieces software. By the time the ACA introduced nationwide penalties for hospital readmissions in 2012, the Pieces team was poised to apply their predictive skills to identify who was more likely to bounce back and do something about it before disaster struck. Amarasingham and his colleagues showed that their algorithms had predictive value for determining if an individual patient with heart failure was at risk for readmission or death within 30 days.[8] This helped the Parkland system create targeted programs and direct scarce resources to people who would benefit from the extra support, all while saving the system half a million dollars in the first year it was implemented, and just in time to be spared as the nationwide penalties for readmissions kicked in in late 2012.[9] By creating a supportive environment for Amarasingham to innovate, the socially minded Anderson had discovered a business case for bridging hospital care with a patient's life circumstances. The team's rigorous studies on improving heart failure[10] management cemented their reputation as national leaders and local problem solvers. Their process was complementary to the work of groups like PACT at Mount Sinai, which were taking an effective but costly approach of assigning skilled caregivers to high-need patients. By the end of 2012, healthcare systems across the country were clamoring for something like Pieces, and a glut of technology companies rushed to market similar-sounding solutions.

Up until this point, Amarasingham had been working within the confines of the public hospital system and within UT Southwestern, where he was trusted. However, in order to invest in the research and development that would expand Pieces, he needed to broaden his efforts. He was supported in spinning off his team's work into the Parkland Center for Clinical Innovation (PCCI)—a nonprofit technology startup that was embedded within the public health and healthcare system. It was all part of a thoughtful organizational structure that Amarasingham had articulated years before while he was at Johns Hopkins, and one that Anderson directly supported by providing him the money for a programmer and direct access to Parkland's EMR. Under Amarasingham's leadership, PCCI was able to recruit the talent it needed; it attracted a multidisciplinary team of nearly 70 people shortly after it spun off.

When healthcare experts speak about bringing the discipline of *value* to how care is organized and delivered, they rarely factor in what environment attracts people to build the high-value systems of the future. Not only had Amarasingham himself declined to join the gold rush of healthcare technology companies after his time at Johns Hopkins, he had also kept others from joining the herd by attracting top "quants" from the nation's best PhD programs, including a brilliant thinker who left a lucrative job in one of New York City's top financial institutions. They recognized the work ahead of them as challenging and nationally relevant. They knew it required not only support from the leadership, but also the bedrock of an institutional mission suffused with a culture of public service—all ingredients that differentiate public systems like Parkland, who have partnerships with strong academic medical centers, from places that merely get the job done.

The PCCI's ethos of technology and business development, all in service of its social mission, is shared by other startups that have grown out of the latest tech boom—like Single Stop USA and Healthify.[11] These new efforts bring refreshed energy and problem-solving capability to longstanding challenges. In turn, they often lead to unexpected breakthroughs in cost and quality for their healthcare system partners, who develop new ways to understand the dimensions of what constitutes high-value care in the process. Rather than being driven by our contemporary moment's laundry list of what constitutes high-value care, they stay focused on defining the social challenges *worth* pursuing, and build the business case along the way. This requires upfront investment and substantial organizational trust.

When Anand Shah approached PCCI in 2012, attracted by its early success with Pieces and growing reputation, he saw firsthand how much lay ahead in the context of the ACA; he also saw just how deep the support for PCCI's mission was within Parkland and well beyond. He immediately recognized that his interest in extending a healthcare system's support more deeply into its surrounding neighborhoods was within reach. Over in Louisiana, by contrast, Fred Cerise was reeling at the hundreds of millions of dollars cut for the care of the working poor and uninsured by Jindal, which the latter stated was necessary to modernize the healthcare system.

ENTER THE NEIGHBORHOOD

Anand Shah joined Amarasingham's team shortly after PCCI was formally spun off from Parkland Health System. He had previously spent time with some of the most forward-thinking groups in US healthcare—the Camden

Coalition, the Center for Medicare and Medicaid Innovation (CMMI), the University of Pennsylvania's Leonard Davis Institute—in search of a way to reconcile his training as an emergency department doctor with the predictable challenges patients faced outside of his domain. The PCCI team's access to Parkland's EHR gave them an unusual advantage that Shah could not pass up. While phrases like "predictive analytics," "big data," and "natural language processing" began percolating up to the hospital executive class in charge of choosing between "population health" software options, PCCI prepared to take on a new challenge: the blindside of the healthcare loop, where patients thrive or languish outside the clinic walls. Anand Shah began calling organizations across Dallas County to find out where PCCI could add value.

Unfortunately, groundbreaking as the Pieces software was, this great technological leap forward alone could not truly incorporate the neighborhood perspective, where the details of how people live and work shape their health. Without modern information systems, a neighborhood's membership organizations, schools, businesses, and places of worship are all in the dark, unable to share in the creation of a truly integrated health system. For the PCCI team to realize their full potential—so that, say, the Salvation Army across the street from Delta's hospital could be in communication with his clinicians and vice versa—they would need to invent ways to share information, protect privacy, collaborate with many other local organizations to create a seamless care plan, and, somehow, pay for it. Each of these dimensions is challenging, obviously. For example, hospitals can theoretically share information with each other through a Health Information Exchange (HIE). However, as Kimberly Gerra, PCCI's Senior Vice President of Strategy, explains, "not all hospitals like to share their data on an open Health Information Exchange because they worry about having patients in their network poached by another system, which leads to more and more proprietary pools of data."[12] This hoarding instinct is exacerbated by the need for most HIEs to support themselves by selling information access. In order to get hospitals and local organizations on board, Shah would have to convince potential participants that the advantages of their technology would far outweigh the risks.

Fortunately, Pieces had a few significant advantages built into its framework. The most significant, in my view, was that all the information about a person was compacted into an intelligent continuity of care document (iCCD), which cleans up hundreds of scattered wisps of information onto one page. The Pieces technology could read the litany of notes of physicians, nurses, social workers, physical therapists, and other caregivers who usually write in specialized, short-hand language and translate them into elegant summaries designed to help anyone reading them make an intelligent decision about what to do next. This meant that information from a range of other organizations and groups across Dallas would also flow into the same, easy-to-read interface. At the same time, Pieces was built to integrate medical and social data into a Dallas-centric data cloud, including information like weather, neighborhood characteristics, and economic data. The real challenges, as Shah states, "are not the technology, but the social, legal and sustainability factors that would make this truly useful for Dallas."[13]

Ultimately, PCCI's vision for their platform aspired to include Parkland's EHR, existing HIEs like the Greater Plains Collaborative (a network of hospitals and providers that covered 6 million people across seven states), more than 400 local organizations, disaster responders, and even the county jail. In order to earn a place at the table among local organizations, the PCCI team recognized that they had to offer solutions to common problems that all of these organizations faced. Instead of taking their prominent position for granted, they leaned on their entrepreneurial instincts and began to investigate the needs of their potential partners.

SHARED SAVINGS

As noted in part 1, most community-based organizations spring up organically to address a specific core need of a small group of people. Generally they are run by passionate individuals who recognize that if they don't act, no one will. These include faith-based groups that have a natural member base, a service that builds a client base, or an advocate group of individuals who actively solve problems and build local expertise in important areas. Many never grow beyond their neighborhood, where they deeply understand the people they serve, their lives, and their needs.

In just about every neighborhood or region there is a small group of people, not easily identifiable, who interact with many neighborhood organizations. John Delta was one of these people. From the perspective of any one of the organizations he interfaced with, it would be almost impossible to tell that he was dangerously healthcare-dependent compared to another client who was momentarily in need of some extra support but otherwise healthy. As Amarasingham realized, not only did Parkland not contact the organizations that regularly sustained Delta; these numerous organizations were also unaware of one another's work with him. Each time Delta needed something specific there was a missed opportunity to really figure out how to help him in a more sustainable way. These organizations lacked the information, but even if they'd had it, they lacked the resources to coordinate their services with potentially dozens of others. When speaking about *value* in healthcare, these connections are rarely factored in.

On the other hand, as the PCCI team found, Dallas County organizations had many common features. Their funders and supporters all required some form of basic outcomes tracking so they could justify continuing their support. Most had a hard time creating metrics to describe their social impact, particularly when they had to stop their usual work to respond to an acute emergency or short-term need. Almost all believed that their own service—whether it be food assistance, nutritional counseling, housing, employment support, disease management, life skills, preventive services, financial education and protection, or senior services—was central to improving the health of their clients. Finally, most had clunky paper records or complicated software to gather, report, and analyze data about the individuals they served. This was far from a hi-tech world, and it was almost inevitable that clients would slip through the cracks as overworked staff struggled to keep their essential service afloat. At the same time, they were concerned about privacy, data security, and limited technology knowledge.[14]

The PCCI team imagined a simple but compelling solution: they would provide easy-to-use client management software called IRIS at much lower cost than the usual options. This, in turn, would connect the organizations to each other and to Parkland through some sort of portal or network that PCCI would build. That was a fine start, but the team also realized that the collective effort of avoiding a dangerous episode of illness requiring hospitalization for a person like Delta was worth a lot to taxpayers who ultimately paid for Parkland to operate, and the savings were worth sharing with organizations who participated in the network. Although the savings in Medicaid spending would be clear, a hospital CEO could rightly be concerned that the program would work *too* well, resulting in not only lower penalties, but also lower revenue from fully paid hospitalizations. The decision to even consider this approach is highly leadership-dependent, which is a reflection of the overall ethos of how a healthcare system is governed. The PCCI had a genuine healthcare system innovation that they could not guarantee would get traction, much less succeed. But they had a strong track record within healthcare *and* across Dallas.

Finally, in 2014, a major $12 million grant from the WW Caruthers Jr. Foundation in Dallas to build a solution, complemented with support from the Commonwealth Foundation to help make it broadly relevant, gave PCCI the boost they needed. Cerise, newly installed as CEO of the Parkland Medical Group, green-lighted their critical support for the project, and the Dallas Information Exchange Portal (IEP) was born. Without further ado, Shah worked with the team to pull together an open town hall for Dallas organizations.

There was strong interest, including from groups who play a role in Delta's life. Of the 24 groups that attended the meeting in July 2014, 18 unique organizations wanted to join the IEP pilot. An organization I am affiliated with in Harlem, City Health Works, was also invited to provide insight from a different national setting. The pilot was a simple proof of concept, with the clear recognition that it would have to learn quickly from mistakes and improve over time. Focusing upon patients like Delta who were high-need, and therefore high-risk for readmission according to Pieces, the IEP pilot set out to improve care coordination across clinical and social service teams. Anytime one of these individuals interacted with an organization in the IEP, this would be recorded using IRIS and trigger an automated payment if, after 30 days, the person was not readmitted to the hospital. At the same time, the analytic capabilities of the Pieces technology, and the elite team behind it, would be lent to measuring and conveying metrics about the quality of an organization's services. Since these quality metrics are not reported anywhere, organizations could use them internally to improve their performance and get better at working with Parkland and other organizations to enhance the lives of individual patients. For example, a high-need patient who lives in a shelter could be supported by an affordable housing organization and job training organization to stabilize her livelihood. All three organizations, if they were on the IEP, would get an automatic payment from Parkland at a level that was meaningful to them while still being substantially cost saving for taxpayers. Because this type of healthcare system and neighborhood integration is so important for the health of Americans if it spreads, Cerise cheered it on even as the Parkland and PCCI team carefully monitored its impact on the public healthcare system's finances and calibrated their approach.

One of the first participants to come on board was the Bridge, an organization that currently serves the majority of Dallas County's homeless population. The very nature of homelessness—with its diverse array of causes and durations—requires a personal, case-by-case understanding of how to bring together multiple services, which is precisely what the Bridge built on its campuses. As the organization's CEO, Jay Dunn, tells it, their approach has been successful, but PCCI offered the potential to really understand how exactly they were currently using resources, and then build predictive models for how to best support someone based upon individual needs.

> Since we opened in 2008, we have had a variety of indicators that are quite positive. Local hospitals are saving money, local jail stays are shorter, and people with behavioral health challenges are two-thirds less costly once they are with us. But our engagement with Parkland and PCCI led us to think about how to best use the overlap of resources with the hospital from the beginning, even starting with transport, on a case-by-case basis instead of in terms of broad populations. How would we develop a customized transition plan, and use our experience to shape a self-learning and self-correcting system? I am sure we will find that we have more gaps than we anticipate, but we are also hoping it will affirm things we do now, and what we learn in terms of challenges, we'll respond to the best we can."[15]

Word about this innovative pilot in Dallas traveled fast, and valid questions have been raised. What about all of the legal arrangements about payments, data sharing, and security? What about the training and support provided to local organizations? How accurately could anyone calculate savings or risk in real time? What about people who were not high-risk or high-need from Parkland's perspective, but who *could be* one day? How much adjustment should take place for more challenging work (the same question that hospitals ask)? Where is the system that allows local organizations to refer to others? What is a fair amount of money to share?

Most of the participants in the pilot program agree that it's impossible to know what the true costs and the true savings are at this point. "I don't think that the current level of financial incentive through PCCI is helpful outside of developing a methodology to figure all of this out," Dunn notes.

"It is easier to raise money independently than do all this work. But that being said, I think the future is some sort of capitated arrangement with healthcare systems, where we all understand our own value in what we are doing for a person."[16]

Compared with the detailed, evidence-based protocols that guide treatment for heart failure, the healthcare system knows almost nothing about the neighborhoods and organizations that support people when they are out of the healthcare loop. We know remarkably little about the right combinations of clinical care with social and economic support that would liberate people from healthcare dependence without pushing them onto overburdened social sector services. The IEP gives us a glimpse into a future of how hundreds of organizations can work collectively to achieve more than the sum of their parts, but it would be a mistake to believe that PCCI's technology, alone, is the solution. Amarasingham and his team know this, and their mission is to channel their expertise toward understanding the existing assets of Dallas neighborhoods; the IEP can play a supportive role. Their willingness to engage in adaptive problem solving by first understanding the scope of the challenge that their patients face enables them to position themselves as *part* of a larger solution, rather than insisting on delivering answers from on high. As a result, when another innovative organization that shares the same problem-solving orientation spreads to Dallas—like none other than Rebecca Onie's Health Leads, which I first encountered back at Harlem—they have a greater chance of building scaffolds of support that endure. Instead of taking a punitive or regulatory role to shape healthcare system design, PCCI, Health Leads, Single Stop USA, and Healthify all represent a new generation of public health organizations that see hospitals as an integral but limited component of improving health in the neighborhood.

Despite the promise these pioneers represent, investments into healthcare system delivery innovation are surprisingly sparse. According to a team from Johns Hopkins, Stanford, Boston Consulting Group, and University of Rochester: "Private insurers ranked last (0.04 percent of revenue) and health systems 19th (0.1 percent of revenue) among 22 industries in their investment in [healthcare service] innovation."[17]

Our minimal investment into discovering how a healthcare system ought to be designed and configured reflects the prevailing assumption that our approach is fundamentally sound, albeit inefficient and wasteful, relatively low-quality, and incorrectly incentivized. This dangerously misguided assumption is exacerbated by contexts like Jindal's Louisiana that are not committed to improving health in all places. As a result, organizations like Health Leads go to healthcare systems where enlightened leadership (or alumni) invites them. Similarly, PCCI is rooted in Parkland's social mission and commitment to Dallas, the same features that attracted Cerise from Louisiana. These places are national bright spots for what is possible when we not only choose to imagine what healthcare ought to be, but have the luxury of leadership that encourages the work of health improvement to pave the way for its financial accounting—*adaptive problem solving* at its finest.

What about neighborhoods across the country that do not have the ideal ecosystem of influential leaders, unique entrepreneurs, and experts to redesign what their local healthcare system ought to do? What about neighborhood organizations in Dallas that may never get connected into the IEP or individuals who may never see a Health Leads volunteer? What about Americans who see a different set of choices that healthcare remains blind to seeing or prioritizing? What about structural disadvantages that no database—even one as sophisticated as Pieces—can address, or healthcare service provision can hope to reconcile?

In a seminal 1996 article, "On Suffering and Structural Violence," the physician-anthropologist Paul Farmer explores what the modifier "structural" adds to the equity equation: "By what mechanisms do social forces ranging from poverty to racism[18] become embodied as individual experience?" In other words, what causes certain individuals, groups, or places to be at systematically greater risk than other groups for suffering? As I asked people I encountered in Dallas why people like Delta become homeless in the first place, I was confronted by a dominant set of social and political narratives that explain where he probably went wrong and what he should do next. Nearly all hinged upon asking where he went wrong, and if he took opportunities to take responsibility for himself.

The dominant social and political narratives that surround people like Delta need to be brought to the surface in order for their unspoken implications for social problem solving to be explored. Doing so requires the proponents of these narratives to confront tensions that otherwise remain invisible. This is why the "cheap talk" between my neighbor and police officers at Clyde Williams's event was so valuable: it surfaced genuine concerns, constraints, and, ultimately, a shared commitment to communicate more closely as issues arose. This is also why visionary organizations like PCCI under Amarasingham, Parkland under Anderson and now Cerise, and Health Leads under Onie choose not to act alone, recognizing that by connecting with hundreds of other organizations, the full scope of a challenge may become visible.

Back in 2009, from the distance of my medical training in Harlem, I had observed Minnesota governor Tim Pawlenty take a similar stance to healthcare reform as Jindal prior to losing the 2011 election to Governor Mark Dayton. Pawlenty had also rejected the ACA subsidies to expand insurance coverage to poor Minnesotans, and like Jindal, simultaneously attempted to cut hundreds of millions from public healthcare funding. Both were toying with quixotic economic plans that aimed to drastically constrain public spending and, somehow, modernize government, without committing to improving health and social outcomes or investing in social innovation and enterprise. Their colleague in Kansas, Governor Sam Brownback, had nearly collapsed his state's economy while significantly cutting funding for education using an even more zealous version of their economic plan.

However, unlike in Louisiana or Kansas, a movement was afoot that contributed to significant social and political change across Minnesota, flying in the face of the draconian executive leadership and ultimately prevailing at all levels of government and the nonprofit sector. In the process, a threatened safety-net system, Hennepin Health, was able to make breakthroughs in how it designed its relationship with the county around it to better serve its people.

I wanted to know how, and so in November 2014 I headed north.

6

Blessed Are the Organized

*Systems awareness and systems design are important for health
professionals, but are not enough. They are enabling mechanisms only.
It is the ethical dimension of individuals that is essential to a system's
success. Ultimately, the secret of quality is love.*
—Avedis Donabedian

GETTING READY TO BE READY

I met my connection to Minnesota, Doran Schrantz, through the Robert
Wood Johnson Foundation Young Leaders group in the fall of 2012. We kept
in touch, and she invited me to attend the Healthy Heartlands gathering
on Veterans Day in 2014 to understand how a unique partnership between
public health practitioners and street-level community organizers had
put inequities in the health of Minnesotans on the map. The initiative was
briefly outlined in a grant description on the W. K. Kellogg Foundation website: "Improve health outcomes for low-income communities and communities of color by engaging and educating select Midwestern organizations
in a process of racial healing and collaboration."[1] The grant was directed
to a group named ISAIAH, which Schrantz led. The Kresge Foundation and
the Blue Cross and Blue Shield Foundation also supported the gathering.
Beyond these hints, I found it difficult to discern what, exactly, the Healthy
Heartlands initiative entailed. In the metrics- and measurement-driven
worlds of public health and healthcare, "improve health outcomes" certainly
sounded conceptually at odds with the amorphous-sounding "process of
racial healing and collaboration."

The title of this chapter refers to the work of the same name by Jeffrey Stout (2012).

And yet as surely as the snow was blowing outside the cavernous Sheraton Hotel banquet hall near Minneapolis–St. Paul, I was swept into the spirit of the Healthy Heartlands conference.[2] The atmosphere was different from what I was accustomed to at healthcare conferences. There were no product displays, posters with graphs, or vacation raffles. People were dressed casually and the spirit was convivial and informal. It took time to get oriented, but there was always someone to provide context. Seated next to me, Rev. Dr. Troy Jackson, director of the AMOS project in Cincinnati, provided a quick history lesson of the groups present while Rex Archer, formerly of the National Association of County and City Health Officials, explained that he had made the drive from Kansas City to "figure out how to get my state unstuck."

Before the keynote speech, Elianne Farhat, a professional organizer, exhorted the audience to share the "recurring truths" that inspired their presence at the event. Some of the truths elicited through crowd sourcing included:

- Populations of high poverty neighborhoods increased by 56 percent since 2000.
- Since 2007 approximately 25 percent of Latino and African American borrowers lost their homes to foreclosure, compared to 12 percent of white borrowers.
- The poorest 47 percent of Americans have 0 wealth.

Farhat had a caveat: "No data without stories, no stories without data!" It was an apt introduction to the speech of Renée Canady, Michigan Public Health Institute's CEO: "We are here to align two fields, community organizing and public health, in a mutual effort to create social justice and health equity."[3] Canady went on, "if you're new to our movement, make no bones about it, community organizing is a field; public health doesn't do community organizing, it does event planning!" As Canady closed, Farhat energetically bounced back, "As we move forward with this work, I want to invite people to stay grounded in their own facts, their own family, but not be content to stay there, but to take on the systems that are making us sick, and build the America that our families deserve."

Everyone seemed focused and engaged, and though I could not yet discern for what, my curiosity was definitely piqued. As the narrative energy in the room steadily and methodically heightened, even I—an undeniable outsider—was emboldened to contribute a story and statistic that moved me at a personal level. On Veterans Day, Ray was on my mind, so I spoke about his grandchildren, who were being raised by a single and struggling mother in an unsafe part of our neighborhood, a context likely to lead to another generation of poor health and limited opportunity.[4] Everyone made it clear that my personal response to what I shared and heard mattered, and there was no use trying to hang back as an aloof expert.

Momentarily out of my element, I looked around for Schrantz, but she was nowhere to be seen. Instead, I had Troy Jackson and Rex Archer on my right and left to serve as my guides. As a community organizer and public health practitioner, respectively, they made an unusual pairing, even more so in the additional company of a physician. During the gathering, both groups blended together, preparing to go back to their respective states and communities, as Canady would say, "to get your people ready to be ready" for opportunities to confront the tensions that kept poor communities and racially marginalized groups from living healthier lives. If this counted as "cheap talk," then it was in preparation for a much larger conversation that they hoped would spill across America's heartland.

HEALTH INEQUITY AND POWER

Earlier in 2014, the Minnesota Department of Health had released a report entitled "Advancing Health Equity in Minnesota," which was co-signed by state departments ranging from agriculture and commerce to corrections and military affairs.[5] The report, spearheaded by Jeanne Ayers, assistant commissioner of health, and Melanie Peterson-Hickey, a research scientist in the Minnesota Center for Health Statistics, "revealed" four critical observations:

- Even where health outcomes have improved overall, as in infant mortality rates, the disparities in these outcomes remain unchanged: American Indian and African American babies are still dying at twice the rate of white babies;
- Inequities in social and economic factors are the key contributors to health disparities and ultimately what need to change if health equity is to be advanced;

- Structural racism—the normalization of historical, cultural, institutional and interpersonal dynamics that routinely advantage white people while producing cumulative and chronic adverse outcomes for people of color and American Indians—is rarely talked about. Revealing where structural racism is operating and where its effects are being felt is essential to figuring out where policies and programs can make the greatest improvements;
- Improving the health of those experiencing the greatest inequities will result in improved health for all.[6]

The fourth observation struck me as a significant shift from a traditional public health and healthcare focus. Instead of viewing health inequities as a deficit that consumes resources, they saw them as a target for investment that leads to *increasing returns*. "Health is not a limited good. Rather than viewing health as something scarce—a resource available only for a few—it is far better to view health from the perspective of abundance—a resource that multiplies the more it is shared. Improving health for those who have the worst health outcomes generates better health for all. Everyone does better together."[7]

To make this case, the Minnesota Department of Health had to define how health is assembled in a way that could truly be relevant for everyone, even people who are not explicitly focused upon health.

The interconnectedness of health among all parts of the community is reflected in the way that health is created. Health is generated through the interaction of individual, social, economic, and environmental factors and in the systems, policies, and processes encountered in everyday life. These include job opportunities, wages, transportation options, the quality of housing and neighborhoods, the food supply, access to health care, the quality of public schools and opportunities for higher education, racism and discrimination, civic engagement, and the availability of networks of social support.[8]

Most notably, the report was startling because it thrust "structural racism," a loaded concept often used by social activists, academics, and faith communities, into the center of a policy report. The language of structures and systems implicitly shifts the weight of addressing complex personal and collective circumstances from individuals to a broader context. Employing this language has complicated effects[9]: it moves conversations away from "racists" as the cause of why minority groups (e.g., Native Americans and refugees) have disproportionately poor health, to systems, but also shifts emphasis away from dominant narratives of how individuals with minority backgrounds overcome their circumstances. The report's upfront confrontational use of "race" and "racism" rather than the proxies of "discrimination" or "injustice," evoked surprisingly strong feelings within me. The systems scientist in me worried about needlessly politicizing a set of observations that could imperil an adaptive problem-solving process. Yet, my time in Dallas had left me with the clear impression that without directly confronting social tensions, we would not even begin to solve the right problems with the right set of perspectives. This is precisely what other newcomers to the Healthy Heartlands gathering worried about as well, and together, we recognized that confronting social tensions is a methodical process that requires a different set of skills than healthcare or public health practitioners are trained in.

Furthermore the examples that the report gave were straightforward and constructive. For instance, when the Minneapolis–St. Paul area was considering a major investment in a light rail transportation system, a simple economic calculation made it obvious that placing stops in rich neighborhoods would allow wealthier people to move around the city and spend their disposable income and contribute to the tax base (higher return on investment). At the same time, it became clear that in the context of the overall budget, cutting three transit stops from low-income, largely minority neighborhoods, constituted a "high-value" decision by policy makers and technical experts. Through a protracted campaign against the default policy narrative of simple cost-benefit analysis, these three stops were preserved. To explain how these transit stops in underserved Minneapolis neighborhoods were saved, the report authors focused on both the goal (equitable public investment) and the process (grassroots community organizing): "If the funding formula of the Federal Transit Administration had not been changed [in response to grassroots community organizing] to take into account community livability along with cost-effectiveness as criteria, the transit-dependent, racially diverse communities along the Central Corridor Light Rail line would have lost, rather than gained, access to transit through this $1 billion public investment."[10]

Using an organizing-based process, within a broader logical framework of equity, the meaning of a high-value public investment necessarily changes. Moreover, growing public awareness of an inequitable decision, one that would further disadvantage poor neighborhoods for decades to come, was channeled into public pressure to change policy. Here and throughout its many examples and analyses, the equity report remained focused upon an overarching solution—that everyone needs the *capacity* to act to change individual and collective circumstances. To break this concept down, people should have the *power* to hold decision-makers accountable, shift how resources, processes, and systems are structured, and build the public understanding and will to act to advance health equity. All of this requires individuals to form relationships and organize as a community to advance their shared aims, which in turn influences how decisions are made and how systems operate in response. Unlike any government report I had read previously, it left me in a state of reflection, curious how it even came to be written in the first place.

The approach the authors took was unusual, as far as government reports go. Instead of simply gathering data, analyzing it, and placing it in prepackaged narratives, the authors invited 1,000 participants from 180 organizations (government and nongovernment) to co-create the narrative that would tell the story that statistics alone cannot. The participants provided 200 dense pages of commentary that shaped the data into an action-oriented narrative that was not preordained, leading the authors to state that its conclusions were "revealed" through a participatory process. Their process also ensured that when the report was released, it reflected voices of people who wanted to take a proactive stance in changing the inequities they observed in their own neighborhoods. Coming from a state that ranks amongst the healthiest in the country, with one of the lowest cost per capita healthcare expenditures, the report was a clarion call against complacency, and a broad call to action.

As state health commissioner, Ed Ehlinger, noted in voicing support of the report at the Healthy Heartlands gathering, "The more power we give to the community, the more powerful we will be as an agency."[11] The gathering steadily reinforced the belief among public health officials—who in many cases felt their influence lagged behind that of healthcare leaders or dwindled in an adverse political climate—that something could be done. At the same time, it required a new set of alliances with community organizers who recognized that health, opportunity, and power were inextricably linked. My fellow participants were energized. So was I.

The conference hall turned into a beehive of activity to facilitate 1:1 conversations. Attendees were encouraged to leave the room with someone they had never met before to get to know them better. Outside the hall, you would never guess that the individuals were newly acquainted, as public health officials and community leaders spoke about their families, values, and what was on their minds. Unlike at a healthcare industry gathering, attendees were not merely networking; they were building enduring relationships. As one community organization leader, Sarah Mullins, put it, "One of the self-interests people have in this work is the desire to transform and to grow. That's often overlooked."[12] Instead of talking about grand strategies or focusing solely upon organizing techniques, leaders imparted the core message that the disciplined and goal-oriented process of building authentic relationships is a path to power in a public arena. For participants at Healthy Heartlands, "authentic" meant the issues that cause tension or discomfort. Whether it was discussion of faith and values in the public arena, or racism and class—these had to be on the table. It was the opposite of polite conversation, where politics, religion, and money are taboo. The participants from Minnesota had seen a path to crisis that would deepen and spread without these conversations, and now, with successes to share as a result of them, they sought to expand their approach.

As a physician from New York, I found the genesis of the Health Equity Report and Healthy Heartlands conference perplexing. I could not imagine how an equivalent document would emerge from the New York State Department of Health, nor envision a broadly participatory process from Bloomberg and Frieden's City Department of Health and Mental Hygiene. So, what were the circumstances that led to a report like this coming to pass, one that ignited a wave of social activism to address its challenges and achieve its goals? At the heart of the approach I saw in Minnesota was *confronting tensions*, which enabled a different type of *adaptive problem solving* from what I had seen in Dallas. I wanted to know more about the authors of the report, and what their relationship was to the groups that hosted and participated in the Healthy Heartlands gathering.

Melanie Peterson-Hickey had been a senior research scientist in the Minnesota Department of Public Health since 2000, with a particular expertise in the health of babies and the measurement of health disparities.

Jeanne Ayers, on other hand, was a relative newcomer to government service—Ehlinger appointed her to the role of assistant commissioner of health in 2011, shortly after Mark Dayton won the governor's race against Tim Pawlenty. When I found out what she had done previously, the juxtaposition of the bold government report and the seamless conference gathering made sense: right before she joined the Minnesota Department of Health, she had led the public health work of ISAIAH, the faith-based community-organizing group that had received the Kellogg grant to host the Healthy Heartlands conference.

Doran Schrantz filled in the backstory and introduced me to ISAIAH.

THE POWER OF ONE

Schrantz herself had joined ISAIAH in 2002 following college at the University of Chicago. After spending some time learning the basics of community organizing practices in Chicago, she welcomed the shift from studying the theory of political and social movements to doing the hard work of collective power-building with groups across Minnesota. She describes her time at the university as a blip in her route from a depressed rural town in Iowa to a "path to discovering [her] *own* power":

> I was not primarily motivated by "helping." I was motivated by my own
> sense of powerlessness and raw anger. And that I believed that we would
> not change anything without being *with* one another rather than *for* one
> another. I was seeking the kind of relationship where we are side by side,
> not one over the other. But rooted in the reality of the world as it really
> is now, not how we wish it was; meaning the place where aspiration and
> values meet the world and something new can happen. That's what build-
> ing collective power, grounded in faith, means to me. And I wanted it for
> *myself*. Otherwise, I would not be able to be one of the leaders of this collec-
> tive enterprise. I would be an "advocate." I am not an advocate. I did kitchen
> table organizing in ISAIAH for 8 years before I was "director." But I was
> being changed by these relationships. I was coming to know myself.[13]

It was Ayers who helped Schrantz see how important power is to realizing public health, all while Schrantz was rapidly organizing larger scales of activity across ISAIAH. Ultimately she was able to steward the strategic action of 100-member congregations (about 200,000 people) that has made a mark across Minnesotan life, policy, and politics.

Ayers, for her part, had taken a very different path to this line of work. Her knack for community organizing was rooted in her rural upbringing: "You wouldn't have electricity unless people had gotten together to agree about electricity. You didn't have to like everybody, but everything got talked through. Someone may agree about paving a road, but not necessarily a fence line. There was tension but things got worked out on the kitchen table."[14] She took a natural interest in public health as an extension of social justice, but was surprised that the professional public health community she encountered was more concerned about a projected shortage of its own numbers than about the health of the constituents they were there to serve. So she drifted until she found ISAIAH.

Neither Ayers nor Schrantz could achieve their broader goals without maintaining their rootedness in the practice of organizing. Schrantz pushed Ayers to see that her interest in public health had to be grounded in relationships that move people, who collectively exert their influence. This key ISAIAH activity is currently led by Marlene Hill, who joined ISAIAH after being awakened to the challenges in her childhood neighborhood: "I came from a poor neighborhood in Mississippi; employment was at 19 percent even before things bottomed out, and I knew I had to learn something about power."[15] Although Schrantz and Ayers are seen as visionary, they view their primary role as street-level organizers, and Hill's work on the ground is at the heart of ISAIAH's approach.

As I learned about what Hill does at ISAIAH, I realized she develops relationships with people at a level that I never have with a patient. Nor is it necessarily akin to a relationship with a friend. Structured 1:1 interactions form the basis of ISAIAH's community organizing discipline (see box 6.1).[16] Especially for people who feel socially isolated, the basic ingredients of a 1:1 interaction are aimed at restoring a sense that they matter, which forms the basis for how they interact with people around them and the issues they care about. The feeling of being part of something larger, especially for people who struggle without strong family or social support networks, or within distressed public housing buildings or unsafe areas, allows them to begin connecting distant and previously unrelated assets in their lives and bring them to a motivated group—in ISAIAH's case, a faith-based congregation. Particularly for Americans who will never be seen as influential

BOX 6.1
Organizing a Movement, One Person at a Time

Credential

Share *what/why* [the organizer] is doing—reaching out and listening to the families of our congregation/community to understand the needs and concerns—with the notion that once we understand the needs of our families, we will try to join together to do something about them.

Reiterate that we are exploring with families—don't know what action we will take—that will emerge from our 1-1 visits with families. What we are clear about is that we need to all walk together if we are going to make meaningful changes in our community.

Focus

Listen to the person's concerns/dreams for the community. Ideally, you will have a deeper understanding of the person's self-interest (what is important to them) by the time you leave.

Ask probing questions

- How long have you lived in this community? How has it changed?
- What are some of your concerns about the community? Are there things you would like to see changed? Why?
- Have you ever tried to address any of the problems in the community? If yes, what was your experience?
- Do you know other people who share your concerns?
- How long have you been a member of the congregation/[community]? Do you participate in any ministries?

Invite

Principle: You only know how real a "yes" is if you give a person the opportunity to say "no." You are not responsible for getting someone to say yes—you are responsible for offering an opportunity to take one step.

Levels of invitation:
1. If the person has energy (passion), invite them to [the organization].
2. If the person is either not very interested/shows little energy/is cautious: ask if we could count on their support down the road if we take action on one of these concerns.

Adapted from PICO Training: 1-1, webpage accessed December 15, 2015, http://www.piconetwork.org/tools-resources/0002.

consumers, because they fall outside the boundaries of an ideal market segment, their role as active citizens rooted in a neighborhood, town, or county gives them a pathway to transforming their lives and environment.

As ISAIAH found through intimate conversations, data about racial disparities was compelling to predominately white groups, but along with data came stubborn narratives of how poor minority groups created their own problems. With a default narrative, what ISAIAH calls the "dominant" narrative, the white congregations of ISAIAH immediately placed data into a story where some people are hard to change and are prone to misfortune of their own volition. ISAIAH realized that without organizing around this central tension, the dominant narrative would remain static, even if the data changed. In the dominant narrative, a demand for more funding for public schools would be met by skepticism that anything more would go to waste, or that too little money was being spent in another category, like healthcare, to justify it. In the path to crisis, a singular focus on fiscal discipline through a narrative of austerity serves a powerful and politically tenable way to pit group against group, sector against sector.

To build self-awareness about their own methods and develop a strategic practice, ISAIAH has partnered with many outside organizations, such as the Kirwan Institute for the Study of Race and Ethnicity at Ohio State University. Their fruitful partnership yielded "Shining the Light: A Practical Guide to Co-Creating Healthy Communities," where Kirwan helped ISAIAH articulate their own dominant narrative:

> The real abundance of the world is only shared by a few. This injustice is upheld by a myth of scarcity. This myth of scarcity builds a world of fear. Because we are afraid we act in isolation, as individuals. Our sense of community erodes and we become even more afraid and more isolated. This perpetuates the myth of scarcity. The world becomes more unjust. We envision a world of racial and economic justice. A world where the abundance of this world is shared by all people, by all creation. We believe that this shared abundance is possible when we are acting as community rather than as isolated individuals. This vision and our faith call us to act out of hope instead of fear.[17]

Through a combination of self-awareness and external partnership, ISAIAH began to not only understand their role in the public arena, but also to become skillful in acting upon it. As Ayers tells it, the combination of her data-driven public health focus and Schrantz's view of community organizing as a strategic practice that could be shared and improved rapidly vaulted ISAIAH from being widely perceived as a small neighborhood organization in the mid-2000s to a powerful regional force that had the capacity to move regional and state-level policy change by 2010. Perhaps the most interesting aspect of the process lies in the fact that ISAIAH didn't start out with a focus on health. Their foray into public health is best represented by their influence on changing the course of public transit investments in Minneapolis–St. Paul mentioned above. Their technical and community-organizing approach represents an advance in adaptive problem solving at the scale of neighborhoods.

BUILDING A MOVEMENT

In 2010, ISAIAH seized upon a multibillion-dollar proposal to build a light rail transportation system through the Minneapolis–St. Paul Central Corridor.[18] To save money, three train stops were slated to be eliminated; all three would serve poor, racially segregated neighborhoods in between wealthier areas. In poor neighborhoods, transit connects people to jobs, reduces the prohibitive cost of transportation, and improves the walkability of the community. It was a clear example of targeted disinvestment in specific neighborhoods resulting from the dominant austerity narrative. The end result was increased restrictive barriers to opportunity and deepened isolation of segregated communities. The "Three Stops Campaign" was part of a larger transit strategy, one that drew upon federal support to ensure equitable implementation. ISAIAH was a core member of eight advocacy, neighborhood, and policy organizations with the specific goal to bring hundreds of people of faith to the effort.

The link to health may not seem obvious at first—certainly not according to the standards set by the healthcare sector, where value formulas are calibrated for individuals. The definition of high-value healthcare does not even extend to the intertwined health of a devoted couple, much less the tapestry of relationships and environmental context they exist within. Public health, on the other hand, is typically handicapped by the opposite problem of scale: their tools for assessing health are not readily adaptable to the vagaries of individual interactions with transit stops and their socio-economic ties to them.

At the same time, healthcare systems are learning the hard way that sick patients in isolated neighborhood conditions tend to grow sicker and more isolated—and therefore more and more costly. In fact, the work of using data-driven red flags to identify "high-need" patients has become a major part of healthcare reform, led by the pioneering efforts of Jeffrey Brenner in Camden, New Jersey. A popular 2011 *New Yorker* article, "The Hot Spotters"[19] put Brenner's findings and terminology in the spotlight, painting a vivid picture of a group of individuals scattered across neighborhoods who are particularly vulnerable to losing control of their life circumstances and becoming healthcare dependent. The healthcare costs these patients incur are enormous, and interest in micro-targeting these particularly vulnerable people and intervening has turned into a cottage industry within the healthcare sector. Interest in this high-need group (colloquially called "super-utilizers" and "top-five percenters") has grown because this small group of individuals consumes 50 percent of a healthcare system's costs.[20] Notably, members of this group are usually low-income, elderly, often members of a racial minority, and unsurprisingly, live clustered in distressed neighborhoods.

The basic premise behind hot spotting is to use cost, health status, and location data to zoom into the broken matrix of support around high-need individuals and to work intensively to patch it up. For the most part, the costs of doing so are much less than the financial consequences of treating them in a hospital. This justifies the provision of a full spectrum of social support, investments into affordable housing, and careful monitoring. Depending upon how their narratives are presented, the world looking in can either see a person who makes poor decisions and incurs extraordinary social costs, or a troubling pattern for groups of Americans who cluster in systematically neglected places. At least for now, the intense focus on identifying high-risk patients heavily skews healthcare systems to design approaches that pull an individual just out of range of a costly downward spiral. Trying to rehabilitate the entire neighborhood where many of these individuals may be concentrated, or supporting their social-support network, is seen as costly, imprecise, and out of scope. As a result, low- and medium-risk people have to surpass a certain threshold of bad life events to access high intensity, micro-targeted services, when a more encompassing but lower-resource approach may suffice. In complement to the "hot-spotter" approach, ISAIAH, under Ayers's direction, saw that an entire neighborhood disconnected from transportation, jobs, and health-care would make everyone more vulnerable.

Ayers introduced the health impact assessment (HIA) as a powerful means to reframe a discussion about financial *costs* to one of restorative *investment* that simultaneously advanced health equity, economic opportunity, and social mobility.[21] The HIA can be defined as "a combination of procedures, methods and tools that systematically judges the potential, and sometimes unintended effects, of a policy, plan, program or project on the health of a population and the distribution of those effects within the population."[22] With this information in hand, the hidden implications of a decision come into view. Bobby Milstein, who develops nationally viable reinvestment strategies that simultaneously improve health and socioeconomic outcomes, mentored Ayers through the process, which ultimately led to a grant from the Robert Wood Johnson Foundation for obesity prevention. It helped that Ayers saw everything related to health as interconnected:

> Faith based organizing and obesity. Doran said we don't do obesity. I said yes we do! We were working on a light rail initiative. I can show you the data that if you have transit, you have less obesity. That was the first health funding that we got. We were part of the Three Stops Campaign. We applied for funding to do a Health Impact Assessment (HIA), but it was hard because there was no recognition of ISAIAH being more than a neighborhood organization at the time. Fortunately, Pew and RWJF came through.[23]

The HIA-driven reinvestment approach is now seen as a useful means to align community development activities with health improvement goals.[24] However, achieving this shift was not simply a matter of changing an accounting table; the process of building a new narrative meant the Central Corridor community had to organize with enough power to influence local decision-making.

As the HIA method gains popularity among healthcare and public health advocates alike, it becomes easy to confuse the technical conclusions of the assessment with the avenues of action that it enables. The "expert" perspectives making those technical conclusions are certainly necessary—even invaluable—when it comes to guiding discussions and defining a collective aim. But focusing solely upon expert-defined interventions eliminates the potential to identify and organize the communities whose lives the HIA is meant to evaluate.

To strike a balance, Ayers invited both experts and community groups to a meeting in the Central Corridor. In a brilliant feat of paradigm shifting, she arranged the room to place the organizing base at the center of the discussion and experts on a side panel, so they would not dominate the conversation:

> That created so much tension because experts felt sidelined. But we were clear about what we were doing. Objective research that isn't informed by values is nonsense: who gets to decide what 20 things we want to study? We cared about job access, transportation access and housing affordability. Ultimately, the experts and Central Corridor neighborhoods selected indicators around those things. They weren't necessarily a likely coalition. The process builds relationships, and lay people gain real expertise.[25]

The ability to embrace, manage, and surface tension consistently emerged as a component of ISAIAH's strategic practice. In fact, it consciously engineers a respectful tension between experts and community groups that anticipates and allows for emotion to spill over the usual bounds of conversation.

Indeed, tensions were running high as Governor Pawlenty focused on fiscal "containment" of spending rather than on the needs of distressed communities. Ultimately, ISAIAH's work was instrumental in bringing poor, racially segregated neighborhoods into the state's broad effort to revitalize the Central Corridor. According to Schrantz, the HIA-based Three Stops Campaign was only a partial success because although the three stops were restored, the broader agenda was stonewalled. ISAIAH could not break through the deep narrative of austerity or scarcity. As a result, they adapted and discovered, through the relationships they had built, that foreclosures were displacing people. This led them to transform the HIA-based campaign into a foreclosure campaign with the same influential base they had built. A year later that led to the passage of the Homeowners Bill of Rights at the state capitol. They had enough power to negotiate with the banks, and preliminary reports indicate the law is having a positive impact. Along the way, their organized base found their path to power and grew substantially as they confronted tensions together. Arguably, it is in the face of antagonistic leadership that community organizing is all the more essential. Significant social tensions are given a constructive channel for frank discussion in an open and public manner that counteracts the shuttering of democratic discourse through intimidation and cutting off access to power.

TILTING THE BALANCE

In 2010, Pawlenty's advantage as an incumbent governor was fading as Mark Dayton rose in popularity with the help of a broad base of well-organized coalitions, including groups like ISAIAH. In the run-up to the election, ISAIAH launched the 10,000 Voices Campaign, with the goal of having intimate house meetings across Minnesota on the topic of structural racism. They had spent the previous decade organizing actions and campaigns like those described above that gave them the confidence to change the course of the governor's election and influence the composition of Dayton's transition team. After Dayton won the election, they invited him to an event at the Minnesota Convention Center along with 1,600 people who had participated in house meetings to share their concerns and priorities. When they planned the event, they had no idea if he would come. Not only did he attend, but his transition team explicitly integrated the people's priorities into his plans for governance. He made the significant appointment of Ehlinger to serve as Minnesota state health commissioner, who immediately invited Jeanne Ayers, whom he knew for her public health work at ISAIAH, to be his assistant commissioner. The balance had tilted.

The group quickly went from a voice in the wilderness to a force in governance, which is precisely when most coalitions lose their coherence and focus as leadership jockeys for power and the culture of government outsiders clashes with long-time insiders. While Ayers pursued the intergovernmental Health Equity Report that would ultimately shake up the system in early 2014, Ehlinger began to spread the concept of data-driven centers for health equity in his role as leader of state health commissioners across the country. Meanwhile Schrantz, continuing in her role as ISAIAH's executive director, extended the reach of their 1:1 strategic practice through a national network of faith-based organizations called the PICO[26] National Network. As Ehlinger, Ayers, and Schrantz were extending their agendas, the ACA was unfolding, and the context was ripe for a redesign of the state's safety-net healthcare systems.

In 2011, the year that Dayton became governor, the state legislature passed two significant healthcare reform measures. The first was to grant two counties (including Hennepin) the ability to design and implement their own healthcare systems, and the second was the ACA-led expansion of Medicaid to low-income Minnesotans. Most regions across the country simply attempt to accommodate the latter without fundamentally revising the architecture of their healthcare delivery. For the most part, healthcare experts believe that large, integrated regional systems will internally reorganize and align themselves to external incentives and consumer demand. This is the basic hope that economists have, as they work with government regulators to guard against monopolistic behavior. On the other hand, there is little proactive work on how a healthcare system should be constructively designed to address the underlying causes of poor health in the neighborhoods it serves. Instead of creating a new way to fly, the process of getting to lower-cost and higher-quality healthcare is thought to be more akin to modifying an existing flight plan.

In 2012, as ISAIAH and its partners began to work with the new state health commissioner to raise the flag of health equity and local decision-making, the commissioners of Hennepin County authorized the creation of Hennepin Health, which took care of many of the region's "high-need" patients living in neighborhoods of concentrated poverty. Hennepin Health combined four organizations that represented healthcare, public health, and social service organizations: Hennepin County Human Services and Public Health Department, Hennepin County Medical Center, NorthPoint Health and Wellness Center (a community health center), and the non-profit, Minnesota-backed Metropolitan Health Plan. As a safety-net system, Hennepin Health would provide care to all of its residents, and by integrating public health, healthcare delivery, neighborhood centers, and healthcare financing organizations it could architect a different kind of healthcare system. These organizations began building a common approach to care that focused upon the integration of "medical, behavioral and social services for an expanded population," in line with the state's effort to extend insurance coverage to all.[27]

One of the powerful consequences of covering *everyone* is that neighborhoods become an effective focus of improvement, particularly for Americans who struggle financially and with poor health, who are regularly failed by hospital-centric care. According to a 2014 *Health Affairs* article, "Seventy percent of the people who enrolled in Hennepin Health in its first eighteen months of operation (2012–2013) are members of racial or ethnic minority groups. Of the 4,884 Hennepin Health members who sought medical care at least once during this eighteen-month period, 90 percent had a diagnosis of mental illness, and 60 percent had a major psychiatric diagnosis such as major depression, bipolar disorder, or schizophrenia."[28] Given the connection between contextual factors and the severity of these conditions, it makes no sense to consider these demographics outside the context of where members live. In light of what Hennepin Health members state they need, it becomes unconscionable: 65 percent reported a lack of social support, 43 percent reported housing needs, and 24 percent reported concerns about drug or alcohol use.[29] By committing to cover everyone in the county, Hennepin had to focus on helping the people it served find stable ways to assemble healthier lives *in their neighborhoods.*

In the Hennepin Health system, instead of getting fees for services rendered, which was the main means of payment prior to healthcare reform, healthcare providers shifted to a value-based system, receiving a lump sum of money per month for the care of their entire population. The natural instinct of healthcare systems that focus on short-term revenue maximization is to figure out how to stabilize high-risk, or "rising-risk," patients with minimal expenditure. This leads them to think, literally, inside their traditional healthcare system box.

Because of the broader social context that shaped Hennepin Health's creation and mission, it used its financial flexibility to invest in high-quality public health and social services, emphasizing primary care. Hennepin invested in care teams—community health workers and care coordinators—who went beyond the hospital, forming a link from the neighborhood to other trained healthcare professionals. They put into practice what Harold Freeman had envisioned, even making his pioneering effort seem limited by comparison. They hired community health workers from surrounding neighborhoods, just as I was beginning to discuss the concept with leadership at Mount Sinai in early 2012. Although the scale of their new neighborhood architecture was modest, it was treated as an integral and necessary element of improving the health of the neighborhood, calibrated to address the needs of vulnerable people who grew sick in pockets of inequity, all while larger social forces worked on improving housing, education, and safety.

One way a healthcare system can understand high-priority neighborhoods is by hiring people from them. Healthcare systems are among the largest employers in their respective regions, and how they use their purchasing and hiring power is central to healthcare system design. Hennepin Health has hired people with local experience as community advocates, housing counselors, and social service navigators. They work closely with data analysts and a host of other healthcare system professionals to customize the services that individuals need outside of the hospital or clinic setting. Preliminary trends are promising—ED visits decreased, primary care clinic visits increased, and the percentage of people who received more complete diabetes care also increased. It is difficult to get patients to notice process-level improvements, but even patient satisfaction increased—to 87 percent. The money that Hennepin Health has saved to date by demonstrating improved health outcomes gets reinvested into a high-potential workforce, which contributes to the local economy.

COMMUNITY ORGANIZING AS HEALTHCARE

Throughout the country, healthcare delivery system infrastructure is most likely to be seen as instrumental to reducing costs and the financial risks associated with illness. As a nation, we continue to take up-and-down economic advice ("do a little more of this, a little less of that"), which lacks insight into what it takes to build a stronger social matrix that gains strength from opportunities to wrap around people who are teetering into trouble. Hennepin Health reflects a sincere effort to push healthcare system architecture to its current boundaries, into a space where dense coalitions can form to turn everyday tragedy into collective opportunity. Like many neighborhood-based organizations across the country that have not traditionally seen themselves as public health or healthcare, faith-based or secular, ISAIAH designated their director of strategic initiatives, Paul Marincel, to work with a national faith-based network, PICO, to focus on health. Marincel remains embedded in ISAIAH and also serves as director of the PICO Center for Health Organizing, where they are experimenting with approaches to bring their strategic practice of community organizing to reimagine a neighborhood health workforce that is capable of authentically bridging the gap between individual needs and neighborhood aspirations.

Marincel's colleagues at PICO recognized that there is a process for fusing the strategic practice of ISAIAH's organizing with the work of healthcare systems across the country that are searching for ways to reach high-need individuals. The basic premise is simple—teach community care teams and healthcare providers a more compact version of ISAIAH's 1:1 practice. Gordon Whitman, PICO's policy leader, reached out to Jeffrey Brenner at the Camden Coalition with this concept, and they formulated a plan to try it out. In 2013, they brought together forward-thinking funders, like the CMS Innovations Center, which were interested in better ways to reach high-need individuals, with traditional philanthropies, like Atlantic, who understood the power of organizing. They devised a way to combine the Camden model—a data-driven process of micro-targeting and supporting high-need patients—with ISAIAH/PICO–inspired organizing principles. To test out their approach, they began implementing their tactic with healthcare systems and the neighborhoods they served in South Dakota, Colorado, Missouri, and Pennsylvania. According to Marincel, preliminary results show "impressive cost savings and health improvements that extend to people around targeted patients."[30] However, the journey Marincel described has been laden with complexity, especially where the data-driven methods of defining high-need individuals are in tension with the strategic practice of organizing, and particularly where it comes to sharing information about personal circumstances with neighbors who could be activated to help. Along the way, Camden and PICO managed to condense the complexity of both approaches into a simpler set of actions that had the potential to spread beyond experts in each area:

> Ultimately, the organizing contribution includes (1) training the providers and their community nursing staff and their care team staff about how to think about how to relate to people in the community through training people how to do 1:1's, how to listen. "Well, the reason I missed my appointments were that, there is no doorbell in my apartment, so I go downstairs and it takes me 45 min to get down and transportation is late, so I go back upstairs cause I can't stand, then I hear a week later they came and I wasn't there." So that couldn't be surfaced until people were trained to sit down and listen. (2) Having community leaders who sit on the care teams, discuss individual clients and the whole process. (3) Coalitions of providers and other stakeholders who are willing to construct a multiprovider system [like Hennepin Health]

for supporting the [high-need patients] so they can improve hospital utilization. The results of coalitions are more mixed right now.[31]

At some point, there may be a carefully constructed clinical trial that shows that the PICO/Camden approach should be added to the national toolkit of health-improvement options. Like the isthmus between two continents and cultures, the worlds of social movements and healthcare currently hang together by these promising threads.

It was the desire to bring these worlds closer that impelled ISAIAH to launch the Healthy Heartlands initiative, based upon the experience it had developed in bringing health and organizing into the same frame. As the Healthy Heartlands conference came to a close, I began to appreciate how much it was, indeed, a gathering, rather than an event. It was years in the making and was suffused with a deep belief that those who joined were together on the right path. When Ehlinger took a moment to remember our nation's veterans and thank those in government service for joining on a day off, I realized that this journey was, indeed, personal for most of the people who were there.

As ISAIAH's journey began to sink in, I became newly aware of the centrality of faith in the stories of others at the gathering, whether they were public health officials or from faith-based organizations. With faith and spirituality at the center of gravity of collective action, social tensions can be confronted as an integral part of technically informed and adaptive problem solving. However, this requires profoundly ethical leadership to orient the social tensions inherent in faithful communities to advance an inclusive social mission.

ETHICAL LEADERSHIP

Before I left Minnesota, I asked Hill what gave Schrantz, a white woman from a rural background, the right to lead a multiracial social movement that confronted segregation and poverty in urban Minneapolis–St. Paul. Couldn't a white woman speaking for minority groups be construed as an extension of structural racism? Possibly, but Hill did not see Schrantz as a white woman. Instead, she spoke about the unique ability Schrantz had to tap into the "joy and visionary place" within people, without pretending that things are not difficult: "She goes [gestures to my heart, pulls something out, and tosses it into the air] look at that!" Her ability to deeply connect with people she meets, to motivate them to confront tensions they feel helpless to change, and to do so within a disciplined collective was at the hilt of her leadership method. The incentive she offered to the people of ISAIAH and its partners was the opportunity to be on the journey to transformative change, through incremental steps that enabled a growing coalition to believe in its power. The intrinsic motivation she harnessed transcended classic financial interests, at least long enough to allow an ethical voice to reframe the terms of day-to-day business.

In my travels around the world, I have seen many faith traditions access their natural reservoir of ethical leadership to constructively confront social inequities: the International Red Cross, Red Crescent, and (officially unrecognized) Red Star of David movement of nearly 100 million people provide humanitarian aid that is often organized at the local level by faith-based groups. What made ISAIAH's approach stand apart, in my view, was their heavy emphasis on 1:1 relationships in the context of an ethical vision—powerful ingredients of a scaffold that both individuals and their community could use to assemble healthier lives, even in unfavorable contexts.

It did not feel at all strange to be a Sikh at a predominantly Christian gathering. Although I had felt comfortable at Ray's funeral service in the church near my home and welcomed by his pastor, the graciousness I felt was akin to being a guest in someone else's home. Perhaps religious advocates would say that something is lost without explicit recognition of the role of a specific faith, but at Healthy Heartlands I felt freer to build upon the work at hand, without feeling like I was trespassing. At the same time, the undertones of faith and spirituality were at once obvious and subtle, seemingly emanating from the personal perspective of participants, rather than from an official stance. Dr. Canady's call to "bring your personal values and beliefs into the room" bobbed in and out of view as data laced with stories permeated workshops that were geared to introducing public health practitioners to the principles of community organizing. To insist upon the right process in the face of rigid technical and financial structures, or seemingly contradictory demands of faith, requires ethical leadership, which is a difficult posture to hold, even for a person like Schrantz.

For instance, Schrantz had barely mentioned that her work was deeply informed by her faith when we first met. Instead, she focused upon the progress ISAIAH has made in moving the needle on transportation decisions, minimum wage, and voter ID laws, particularly where they disproportionately would have impacted low-income Minnesotans. She only mentioned the word "congregation" after being asked how so much had been accomplished in the span of a few years. Ayers, who was plucked from ISAIAH into government when the current governor Mark Dayton was elected in 2011, was quicker to explain how integral faith has been to her journey:

> I grew up in a Catholic household that was deeply justice oriented; I was
> part of a church that had not mentioned the word in over 15 years, but I did
> not feel that it was right to migrate to a more liberal church with a liberal
> priest, so I gave my church 6 years to bring some conversations and tension
> with the help of ISAIAH . . . I went into public health because of my faith. It
> is basically secular Catholicism. That was a revelation: the concept of being
> one person that I don't have to segment. There is a lot of power and strength
> when you understand who you are, the relationship of what you want
> from the world. I realized that people who were working on transportation,
> education, and jobs were working on health but they didn't know it. How
> powerful would it be if they did?[32]

Schrantz's approach is different, simultaneously steady and searching, rooted in a tough childhood in Iowa where she witnessed the collapse of her regional farming community: "It was terrible for their financial security, but, more devastating, it was terrible for their hearts and minds."[33] In her words and actions, it is easy to see the blend of her world-class education coupled with the practice of building transformative relationships with people who comprise ISAIAH and its partner networks:

> We [ISAIAH] are faith based, and it is our primary identity. In a conference
> setting, we don't always lead with it, however, it is our identity in a public
> arena. The health conversation taps people's faith very deeply. In a Christian
> tradition—we are one body that is connected, in contrast to the lie that we
> are fundamentally separate—provides a pathway to overcome difference
> and pain. For me, it is the only hope. There is so much that tears us apart.
> People's faith provides them some framework that is not an American
> partisan framework, that isn't rooted in American racism, if you can tap it.
> The health-faith-power conversation is the conversation about transforming ourselves, transforming people. People are nervous about church people

everywhere. They have a bad rep[utation] for good reasons. There has been a misuse and abuse of religion in American politics. We are careful about that. We are trying to bring in healing, expanding the discourse, and if you don't come from a religious perspective it can be useful to have people operating out of faith.[34]

I was struck by her last comment, "useful to have people operating out of faith." Certainly in my scientific training and work in economic development, it was difficult to make the stepwise, evidence-based, and rigorous arguments that could change a dominant narrative. As a result, adaptive problem solving that takes place without appealing to more intuitive principles—compassion, love, and faith in our collective ability to build a healthier neighborhood and nation—simply leads to increasingly clever and opaque solutions to problems that displace what truly ails us. The idea of *confronting tension* is encapsulated in the structured 1:1 format, because we have to discover what keeps each of us back from living a healthier, more joyful life. As 1:1s build into organized coalitions, we feel more ready to confront social and economic tensions that hold our neighborhoods back from being healthier places. Although the faith-based underpinning and organizing techniques were new to me, they have long enabled neighbors to coach their neighbors into setting and achieving their aims; as a coalition of individuals grows from this common experience, it builds power to redesign systems and structures around it that have contributed to adversarial contexts. As this takes place, the possibility that any one individual can *assemble a healthier life*, upon a scaffold of support that grows with them, becomes more likely.

As a result of my time in Minnesota, I saw signs of a coaching culture all around me, including in Harlem.

7

Coach Culture

*Eventually everything connects—people, ideas, objects . . . the quality
of the connections is the key to quality per se . . . I don't believe in this
"gifted few" concept, just in people doing things they are really interested
in doing. They have a way of getting good at whatever it is.*
—Charles Eames

GABE

Whether or not healthcare systems wish to acknowledge it, our health is shaped and maintained outside the clinical environment, in the realm of our daily existence. Consider the true story of a little boy named Gabe, whose rare condition has had a cascading effect on nearly every aspect of his life. His mother, Cristin Lind, drew a picture of the 70 people clustered in different groups who were integral to the care of her child (see figure 7.1). Her son is at the center of her drawing. It is hard to imagine one system that could be capable of seeing Gabe's essential needs in the same way that his mother does. Nor does Lind argue that any one entity or system should. However, the energy it takes her to make her son's life a healthy one is staggering. Countless Americans who are capable of working do not do so in order to focus on stabilizing their family's lives—51 percent of people who are non-employed cite health problems.[1] Although Gabe's relationship with healthcare is unusually complex, Americans regularly experience uncharted variants on the same theme of feeling unsupported and lost.

Cristin Lind's family eventually moved to a place that had a better support system. What if Lind had been able to find the missing layers of support that America needs to build right in her community?

FIGURE 7.1

Gabe's Care Map

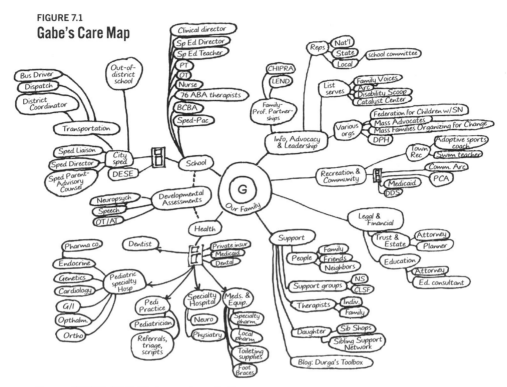

Source: © 2014, Cristin Lind, www.durgastoolbox.com.

QUALITY OF CONNECTIONS

Today, most healthcare systems across America recognize that they must play some active role in coordinating the services an individual receives, whether in the context of multi-specialty cancer treatment or post-hospital care for high-need patients. Multiply the number of people a healthcare system sees in a year by the combination of services a person needs or desires. With the dizzying challenge of making trillions of connections a year, the idea that a healthcare system's sole focus should be on delivering clinical services seems misplaced.

In an age dominated by technology, a problem of this nature screams for a technologic solution. Today, healthcare systems are hiring thousands of care coordinators. Their jobs remind me of old telephone operator services, where workers manually connected phone lines as Americans patiently waited to speak with each other. There were static-ridden lines, dropped calls, and miscommunication. However, a technology that would try to simply automate the work of a care coordinator can only do what it is told; we are far from the point where we can automate the discoveries about a patient that would replace today's unreliable interactions.

Despite our healthcare sector's costly efforts, communication is poor, connections are missed, coordination is cursory, and the quality of interactions with people is low to begin with, even before a person's context is taken into consideration. For a kid like Gabe, healthcare is clumsy at best, a nightmare at worst. As the pioneers in Dallas and Minnesota know, coordination without adaptive problem solving or the ability to confront tensions that individuals and neighborhoods face is doomed to inefficiency and, ultimately, failure. Without a means to systematically improve the quality of each and every connection—between people, and between people and healthcare systems—neither incentives nor regulation are useful. Healthcare systems need a health coach.

In his article "Personal Best," Atul Gawande offers a cogent explanation of what an ideal coach does: "Good coaches know how to break down performance into its critical individual components. In sports, coaches focus on mechanics, conditioning, and strategy, and have ways to break each of those down, in turn."[2] Good coaching requires observation, listening, and guidance to transform a human instinct—like Lind's desire for Gabe to live a healthier life—into the skillful ability to co-create a health system that works. With or without technology, a systemwide coaching function happens one connection at a time.

In my travels in Africa and Asia, I have encountered community health workers (CHWs) nearly everywhere. Their roles varied widely. To help meet the health needs of their neighbors they served as the glue that held together neglected rural health systems, acted as MacGyver-like problem solvers who fixed latrines and treated malaria, and became forceful community advocates in policy settings. In my travels across the United States, I have noticed that CHWs exist in small pockets, like in Arkansas's Community Connector Program,[3] but their presence grows as evidence shows that they are an important piece of healthcare. The American Public Health Association defines a community health worker as follows:

> a person who is a trusted member of and/or who has an unusually close understanding of the community served in the delivery of health-related

services through either working directly with providers or their partner organizations. This trusting relationship with the community enables community health workers to serve as a liaison between health and social services and the community to facilitate members' access to services and improve the quality and cultural competence of services delivered. Community health workers build individual and community capacity by increasing health knowledge and self-sufficiency through a range of activities such as outreach, community education, informal counseling, social support and advocacy.[4]

Most people know someone in their life who naturally does many of these things. Formal recognition and investment in their social role means that their skills can be cultivated, improved, mastered, and remunerated. They also play an integral role in assembling a health system that truly works for the people they serve. One of the reasons why there are so many names for community health workers (for example, *promotoras*, *accompagnateurs*, health coaches) is that their emergence usually stems from some pressing issue or problem that calls for a local advocate—an organic process that is anything but standardized. Over time, it is only natural that the community health worker's role, relationships, and expertise evolve with experience. Many purists insist that their training remain limited to community advocacy and do not encourage them to acquire fluency and skills in healthcare sector processes. But circumstances too often demand such fluency for the purist approach to make sense. In Alaska, for instance, community health workers play a crucial role as extensions of the clinical system where there are few doctors to cover a vast frontier. Pediatricians Mark and Sarah Redding spent years working in the Alaskan frontier, then translated what they had learned to Ohio, where they placed community health workers in the context of paid, results-based, and integrated pathways of care coordination between healthcare systems and neighborhood organizations and agencies.[5] The pioneering work of the Reddings places community health workers in the loose concept of a community health hub, which is envisioned to be rich with neighborhood partnerships and a focal point for sustainable, neighborhood-level health financing. While their particular approach is gaining traction and national recognition, there are hundreds of other notable efforts to make CHW-based initiatives endure, and each approach can claim a unique philosophy and set of goals. All are working on a common question: What is the role of neighbors helping neighbors to assemble healthier lives, which can directly enhance the quality of healthcare connections to it, and within it?

Nearly all community health worker programs focus on developing long-term relationships with the people they serve, although they vary considerably in how they do so. One commonly used technique is called motivational interviewing (MI). The approach was popularized by a pair of American and British clinical psychologists, William R. Miller and Stephen Rollnick, who have taken pains to convey that the spirit of MI (see box 7.1) is more important than the specific techniques: "Motivational interviewing is a way of being with a client, not just a set of techniques for doing counseling," which in turn allows you to "become a helper in the change process and express acceptance of your client."[6] Importantly, the MI approach begins with the premise that we may feel ambivalent about changing our context or committing to new goals. Reflective listening and affirmation of a person's context yields "expressions of problem recognition, concern, desire and intention to change, and ability to change," which can be selectively

---

BOX 7.1
The Essence of Motivational Interviewing

1. Motivation to change is elicited from the client and not imposed from without.
2. It is the client's task, not the counselor's, to articulate and resolve his or her ambivalence.
3. Direct persuasion is not an effective method for resolving ambivalence.
4. The counseling style is generally a quiet and eliciting one.
5. The counselor is directive in helping the client to examine and resolve ambivalence.
6. Readiness to change is not a client trait but a fluctuating product of interpersonal interaction.
7. The therapeutic relationship is more like a partnership or companionship than expert/recipient roles.

Adapted from Stephen Rollnick, Ph.D., and William R. Miller, Ph.D., "What Is Motivational Interviewing?" *Behavioural and Cognitive Psychotherapy* 23 (1995): 325–34.

reinforced so an individual becomes conscious that he or she is in a process of change.[7] As compared to the structured 1:1 approach that ISAIAH uses, which focuses upon what an individual is willing to do with or for others, the MI approach focuses upon coaching individuals through a process of discovering how they can authentically engage themselves in a change, although they may not know how.

During my 12 years of post-college biomedical education, patient interactions were portrayed as either information exchanges or occasions for making joint decisions; there was little emphasis on creating an enduring relationship as a primary goal. By not taking advantage of this interaction, physicians lose an opportunity to become effective and welcomed neighborhood advocates, and patients lose an opportunity to be central actors in healthcare redesign. While physicians prepare for more time-pressured patient encounters where their role is seen as diagnostic, management-oriented, and interchangeable with their colleagues, community health workers are on the frontlines of developing a high-quality connection with their neighbors and their healthcare systems.

The home environments a community health worker enters are strikingly different from one another. Some homes have kids running around; others are quiet and have had no visitors for years. One apartment is a maze of old magazines and boxes in all directions with piles of dirty dishes and pet food spilled on the floor. In another, the CHW must remove her shoes before entering the immaculate rooms and finds medications carefully labeled in a box. In one home a TV blares or neighbors shout. In another, complete silence reigns. There is no sure-fire protocol for how she will create a zone of focus for the encounter, no consistent checklist for understanding an individual's system for living. The MI techniques are employed to elicit her client's goals: someone may be initially uninterested in "better diabetes control" but may be quite concerned about her parents' or children's health. The community health worker finds opportunities to reframe "better diabetes control" in the language of a person's own motivations and sources of ambivalence. This technique helps clients to see that they *do* have wide-ranging health goals, even if they think about them in very different ways. In the process they may discover their personal system, and even the principles that underlie *why* they consistently make certain decisions. When MI is combined with tailored education that is directly relevant to their own goals, clients not only become skilled at setting and achieving goals, but also share what they learn with friends and family. Sometimes a coach can also be a peer with personal experience living with a similar health condition, as one community health worker described in an encounter with one Ms. T.

> About 6 years ago, I was about 300 lbs. and I had the lap band surgery. [After,] I was going through a period where I couldn't eat, and I was reject-ing healthy food, and all I wanted was sweets and candy, and anything else was just coming up; I would vomit, it was just horrible. [My client,] Ms. T was telling me all of these things [her similar experiences] and I asked her if she had the lap band surgery and she said, "Yes! How did you know?" and it was just an immediate connection . . . "My doctors haven't even been able to figure it out." I told her that her lap band was too full and she had to get some saline removed so she could eat and intake more, and be healthier . . . She immediately told her doctor and when she removed the saline she was able to eat what she was supposed to, and that was really memorable.[8]

Although clients and their community health workers don't always share similar life experience, a gifted CHW can catch personal details about whomever she is speaking with and connect on this basis. Personal rela-tionships the CHW forms with doctors and staff at a primary care clinic enhance this sphere of knowledge. Small discoveries people make that could be important for someone else can be mentally cataloged and saved for later: how a neighbor bypassed an onerously bureaucratic process, or a physician's view of how the clinic *actually* operates.

CITY HEALTH WORKS

Just prior to starting residency at Mount Sinai, I had chaired the One Million Community Health Worker Technical Taskforce, which provided guidance for how to deploy a new generation of community health workers to serve as the connective tissue between communities and struggling rural clinics across sub-Saharan Africa.[9] This eventually turned into a multicountry cam-paign.[10] As I immersed myself in clinical training, it was easy to lose sight of how any of this work was related to health in Harlem. Donya Williams, the public health practitioner in charge of the Healthy Bodega Initiative de-scribed in chapter 4, helped me recognize that despite the density of health-care and public health interventions that were being deployed in Harlem, they were often thwarted by poor connectivity. Shortly after Williams left the NYC Department of Health, a young social entrepreneur named Manmeet Kaur met with her for different reasons: Kaur was working on building a social enterprise to improve the entry-level health-related jobs in underserved neighborhoods, an area of interest she had pursued for a decade, and was looking for someone to help her launch it. (Full disclosure: Kaur is my wife.) They made an ideal team, and I was eager to share what I had learned abroad as a strategic advisor. Their organization, City Health Works, aimed to train community health workers, which they called "health coaches," in MI techniques to support their neighbors in improving chronic disease management and organizing them to overcome neighborhood-level barriers. In their preparatory work,[11] they realized that their coaches would have to be relentlessly focused upon improving the quality of connections, not only from healthcare systems to their patients, but also for how their neighbors assembled a larger array of support and services. In late 2012, Mount Sinai agreed to pay for their services in the context of their accountable care organization (ACO) and Patient Centered Medical Home (PCMH), along with philanthropic support from the Robert Wood Johnson and Robin Hood Foundations. They found a mentor in Angela Diaz, who grew up as a struggling teen in the neighborhood and now leads the largest Adolescent Health Center in the country, where she was once a patient.[12] Since Diaz worked with teens, she was intimately familiar with the idea of meeting her patients where they were comfortable and in ways they trusted.

City Health Works's offices are located in the Oberia Dempsey[13] Multi-Service Center, which is "a 'one stop' social, health, educational, recreational and neighborhood service center whose purpose is to bring the local services and activities close to those in need."[14] The building is a former public high school, and the rooms that City Health Works has furnished are a bright contrast to the NYC Department of Probation's Harlem Neighborhood Opportunity Network (NeON) offices located across the hall. The Dempsey Center is within the Harlem Children's Zone area, a few blocks away from the district's congressional offices, and a few minutes' walk from Sylvia's, a touristy soul food restaurant, and the pricey Red Rooster eatery. Nearby one can see the legendary Apollo Theater's signage on 125th Street from the door of a busy Starbucks on Malcolm X Boulevard. The famously bustling intersection boasts the fruits of economic development and rapid gentrification, including a high-end Whole Foods grocery store. On the same street, fast-food stores happily consume the disposable income of Harlem's residents, many of whom pay exorbitant fees to cash their paychecks at storefront services because they don't have a bank account. Old-timers tell me that just a few decades ago you could walk for blocks in Harlem without seeing a soul, and even today people who have long since migrated to the suburbs raise their eyebrows in disbelief at the thought of raising a family in the neighborhood.

Kaur grew up in Queens and studied in New York City before she left the country to work on innovative approaches to health and livelihoods in India and South Africa. In South Africa, she helped a group of HIV-positive individuals create a yogurt business at Mamelani Projects,[15] a nonprofit that provided peer-based health education. She found that the peer-based model produced a sense of confidence that led the group to gain economic independence through creating their own livelihood. It simultaneously produced a fundamentally different relationship to their health. From Kaur's experience abroad, she saw that the active ingredient of an adaptable, neighborhood-based health system resided in the confidence and dignity that peer-based workers helped create.[16] In Kaur's previous work, at NYU's Brennan Law Center, she had seen firsthand how workers in poorly regulated healthcare jobs, like home-health aides, were treated by healthcare systems and the social service agencies that hired them.[17] Rather than viewing community health workers as a low-cost neighborhood extension of the healthcare system, or marginalized neighborhood health advocates, Kaur saw health coaches incorporating and rising above both roles. City Health Works's foundational premise is that investing in the professional development of coaching skills among all—staff and members—is its means of learning where its clients' individual health goals can activate neighborhood-level action and healthcare systems change. Because Mount Sinai had money to invest in new approaches to population health through their ACO and PCMH program, City Health Works gained access to their EHRs and developed a close relationship with clinical leaders who were rethinking how primary care should be delivered, similar to how PCCI is related to the Parkland system.

For Williams, the opportunity to build City Health Works from the ground up was a way to address what she felt was missing in the Healthy Bodega Initiative. She saw the development of high-quality jobs for health coaches, who in turn could help their neighbors construct healthier lives, as a means of aligning with the neighborhood's aspirations, rather than with the mandates of healthcare or public health alone. Her focus remains on the organization's operations, which enables it to support coaches as they move throughout the neighborhood and maintain seamless relationships with dozens of social agencies and community organizations. Jamillah Hoy-Rosas, who leads the practice of Health Coaching and Clinical Partnerships, joined Williams and Kaur. As a registered dietician, public health practitioner, and certified diabetes educator, she brings the know-how to interact with the fast-paced clinical world. All three of the organization's leaders consider their chief roles to lie in supporting the coaches' discovery of how best to help their neighbors, using what they learn to build a sustainable business model and continuously identify areas of improvement.

The City Health Works coaches join forces to find the ideal match between neighbors and the unique skills of a coach—a collaborative and adaptive referral system—one that is rarely seen in clinical and public health settings. In getting to know two City Health Works coaches in particular—Norma Melendez and Evelyn Cruz—I have benefited from a privileged view of how interpersonal styles can differ among coaches, and why a diversity of coaching styles is a source of strength, rather than a threat to standardization, for City Health Works.

When Melendez speaks to you, she focuses intensely on your expression, allowing her to intuitively sense when you are getting lost and loop back around to fill in a missing detail. She knows East Harlem and its people intimately. Her mother died when she was five and her grandmother, who raised her, developed debilitating Parkinson's disease when she was in her early teens, leaving Melendez with the challenge of taking care of herself in a tough neighborhood. Somehow, she got through school, found jobs to sustain her along the way, and built a support network that she could genuinely trust. Melendez realized that she *enjoyed* figuring out how the neighborhood and its supporting organizations *really* worked. She is curious about how people find their way and collects tips that she eagerly shares with whomever she meets: "I've relied on hundreds of people to be a resource for me, and I want to be a resource for people I meet."[18] The practical knowledge she has, for example about how to make sure your New York City affordable housing lottery application doesn't get lost or ignored, should alarm its administrators, who rarely see the haphazard workflows that her neighbors must master to secure basic necessities like safe housing. She spent years working in homeless shelters, with clients who access nearly every possible public and social service. She was regularly dismayed that each of the dozens of services she had to interact with, including the healthcare system, simply cared about their own process measures, rather than seeing each other as part a goal-driven neighborhood system of helping clients assemble a healthier life, which includes the right level of interdependence we all need on an ongoing basis.

Melendez's ability to rapidly connect with nearly anyone as a peer is a unique strength; it is distinct but complementary to Cruz's style. Cruz is a few decades older than Melendez, and loves taking on the role of a tough grandma, one of the neighborhood's old-timers. She grew up in a public housing tower similar to Ray's, and she paints a vivid picture of how strict she had to be as a mother to ensure that her kids not only got educated, but got home safely and stayed out of trouble every single day. "You have to create a system that works for your family and your neighbors, and then stick with it," she recommended. "You can't have eyes everywhere, and you need your neighbors to know your system so they can help out when you're not there."[19] Her personal journey with asthma, diabetes, and breast cancer made her realize that ultimately your methods and outlook shape your health:

> So what I think has saved me is determination, faith, but also my method of seeking out knowledge. If I don't think what you're giving me is credible information, I'll get a second opinion. That saved me. When I was diagnosed with type II diabetes—I was just given a list of foods to avoid. I needed to know more—because what I found was that when I followed the diet my sugar plummeted—so I started keeping a log and taught myself. . . . Diabetes is diet related; the first thing they tell you is what you can't do. I don't think that works, especially when people are economically challenged. . . . Instead if you take a positive role: let's turn this into what you *can* do, not a negative, but a positive thing.[20]

Even though Cruz and Melendez perform essentially the same function at an individual level, they reassign clients whom they think would be a better fit with another coach, allowing the team to tightly connect with Harlem's diverse population. Whereas Melendez came to City Health Works through STRIVE International, an East Harlem–based organization that supports job training and paths to economic self-sufficiency, Cruz took a more accidental route when she met an employee of City Health Works at Corbin Hill, a local community supported agriculture (CSA) business. Since each coach came to the organization through different outreach processes to ensure a diversity of experience with the neighborhood, there needed to be a common professional development experience, so over time, their neighbors would know what to seek through them. At their weekly Wednesday morning case review with Hoy-Rosas, Director of Health Coaching and Clinical Partnerships, and Williams, Director of Operations, the team shares progress, challenges, and techniques to coach their clients. At the same meeting, Hoy-Rosas and Williams make sure that the coach-client goals are well defined, that the coaches are equipped with the best methods to support them, and that connectivity to neighborhood social services and the healthcare system remains strong. City Health Works emphasizes continuous quality improvement, a reflection of Kaur's study of W. Edwards Deming's view of an organization as part of a larger coaching system that is constantly evolving:

> The prevailing style of management must undergo transformation. A system cannot understand itself. The transformation requires a view from outside. . . . The first step is transformation of the individual. This transformation is discontinuous. . . . The individual, transformed, will perceive new meaning to his life, to events, to numbers, to interactions between people. Once the individual understands the system of profound knowledge,[21] he will apply its principles in every kind of relationship with other people. He will have a basis for judgment of his own decisions and for transformation of the organizations that he belongs to.[22]

At these Wednesday meetings, Hoy-Rosas leads a review of how the coaches are doing with their clients, with all staff present. They take confidentiality seriously and the growing list of curious visitors—from insurance companies, neighborhood organizations, city officials, healthcare systems, and potential supporters—are not allowed to attend this particular session. In the reviews, a client's personal circumstances give context to his or her clinical challenges: a divorce; a foreclosure; the death of a loved one; a job lost; depression; anxiety; the resurfacing of an old mental or physical trauma; a new "bad habit" within the family; illiteracy; confidence, slowly whittled down or shattered quickly. Sometimes good opportunities arise: a new job; a new love; the return of an old friend; the departure of a bothersome presence; new and better housing. Even with good news, fragile systems of maintaining personal health may adapt poorly in the face of abrupt change. On the foundation of a shaky present, planning for the future can feel like a luxury. For someone who is teetering on the verge of poor health amidst a range of other challenges, more pressing matters easily displace the daily monotony of taking a pill or scrupulously following a clinical recommendation.

The Wednesday morning meetings focus on the hard work of *assembling health* in the neighborhood, work that we all must do with or without support. Even in the presence of structural inequities or complex illness, the work of remaining on a steadily healthier path requires constant effort and attention; there is no cruise control for any of us, even those naturally endowed with excellent physical health. At critical moments when we find ourselves stressed and stretched thin, even seemingly good health can fall apart. In healthcare sector language, experts often reference "gaps" in care. Are the gaps small, awaiting a specific fix? Or are they enormous, beyond the capabilities of any system to fix them acting alone? On Wednesday mornings, these questions are not academic: they define how the organization acts and what it builds, informed by the steady insights of coach interactions with their clients, their neighbors. Instead of arriving at one consensus position, the entire team, from the coaches to the executive director, listens to the same stories and incorporates their very different answers to each of these questions into their subsequent interactions.

As the team's link to clinical partners, Hoy-Rosas logs into the EHR databases of participating healthcare systems to read the notes and lab results of clients who have authorized City Health Works to do so. She identifies issues that can be more effectively addressed outside of the clinic setting, regularly speaks with the clinic's care coordinators about client issues that may need more urgent attention, and proactively communicates with clinicians about quality issues that emerge from client concerns. Even though City Health Works has a "starter kit" of ways to interact with clinical systems, such as how a care coordinator interacts with Hoy-Rosas for weekly case reviews, these protocols are co-designed with clinical partners to fit the highly variable ways that primary care and population health teams operate. Big medical centers like Mount Sinai or Harlem Hospital are organized in substantially different ways from neighborhood clinics that are part of the large Institute for Family Health network, or part of historic neighborhood organizations like Settlement Health or Boriken. Their information systems communicate minimally, if at all, and people in the neighborhood regularly bounce between them. Hoy-Rosas addresses a neighborhood-level gap in "care coordination" between multiple healthcare systems that care for individual City Health Works clients. As different clinics interact with the same neighborhood-based organization, City Health Works, it reduces variation and redundancy in how they communicate and connect with their patients in the neighborhood setting.

At the Wednesday morning meetings, Williams's focus is consistent with her previous work for the Healthy Bodega's initiative: ensuring that her team is motivated and interacting fluidly with dozens of neighborhood partners who can help to address client challenges that relate to social and financial hardships. From the perspective of the social service organizations, faith-based organizations, and city agencies, Williams is a bridge to understanding how healthcare systems work financially and operationally. She is constantly looking for ways to streamline the process of interacting with dozens of organizations, determining who may be able to help their clients in ways that fit with the tailored goals that City Health Works coaches identify in collaboration with their clients and their clinical care team. Instead of trying to deal with all of a person's challenges at once, coaches work with their clients to prioritize a litany of potential goals, which helps Williams focus upon which neighborhood partners City Health Works should build relationships with first. Most importantly, she provides extensive feedback to partner organizations on the experience City Health Works clients have, how they can be improved in the future and better targeted to achieve measurable goals. For instance, the New York City Health Commissioner, Mary Basset, had seen the impact of community health workers in her years of work in Sub-Saharan Africa, and she wanted to bring them into the mainstream. Her staff spent a considerable amount of time learning from City Health Works before launching its own effort, which focuses on obesity and diabetes management in the neighborhood's public housing projects. In return, City Health Works has considered developing a more comprehensive approach to public housing buildings, where many of its clients live. In this way, a coaching culture enables an entire ecosystem of supporting organizations to build higher-quality connections with their clients, shifting their job from assembling many scattered pieces of support toward the life goals that they are at liberty to define.

NEIGHBORHOOD CHANGE AGENTS

Insights from the Wednesday morning meetings yield other, previously undetected avenues for neighborhood advocacy. When City Health Works coach Leny Rivera heard about a movie theater that had called police on a diabetic man who'd brought strawberries to the film to keep his blood sugar levels in check, she was incensed.[23] She and her fellow coaches complained about the theater's policy. The theater yielded. Multiply this degree of change by a hundred small improvements, and not only does the neighborhood become an incrementally healthier place to be, but neighbors also begin to recognize that their collective efforts are meaningful. These small victories, in Renée Canady's words, get people ready for being ready, for a time when more complex challenges inevitably fall upon them.

By design, City Health Works expands its service area in the shape of the congressional district, in recognition that many issues that affect the neighborhood require political leadership.[24] The coaches hope that successors to Congressman Rangel will recognize that improving the health of the neighborhood isn't just a matter of breaking new ground on healthcare facilities or supporting a legislative priority. Equally important is the problem solving that emerges from the process of engaging people at the street level.

The unique challenges each client presents constitute fresh opportunities for City Health Works to recognize patterns that can be translated into organizational-level goals. For example, because of the strong rapport that coaches build with clients, details of personal traumas often surface, revealing much higher levels of depression and anxiety than originally anticipated. This has led the organization to integrate "trauma-informed care" and a "collaborative care model"[25] for mental health as part of its system of engagement.

Although the coaching approach differs substantially from the 1:1 organizing methods that ISAIAH employs, both interactive methods enable the entire organization or movement to change its focus to meet the most pressing needs of its constituents. Doing so builds greater trust and solidarity both between community members and between clients and coaches. Clients, in turn, are more inclined to improve upon their own coping systems when they are able to access a coach they trust to guide them.

Consequently, among City Health Works's first 200 clients, coaches helped avert 30 unnecessary ED visits,[26] all because clients called their coach first, who then urgently informed their clinical care team, who then arranged for the clients to be seen in a primary care setting instead. The results were beneficial for all involved, in terms of cost, quality of patient experience, and health outcomes.[27]

CONNECTING PEOPLE TO PRIMARY CARE

Much of the success of City Health Works will depend on how assiduously Mount Sinai continues its quest for higher-quality connections between its systems and the populations they serve. In 2007, the Patient Centered Medical Home (PCMH) care model was formally described in a joint statement by multiple medical organizations—the American Academy of Family Physicians, American Academy of Pediatrics, American College of Physicians, and the American Osteopathic Association. A year later, healthcare leaders Don Berwick, Thomas Nolan, and John Whittington imagined the existence of an "integrator" organization with five basic responsibilities: "partnership with individuals and families, redesign of primary care, population health management, financial management, and macro system integration"[28] fitting into a geographic area. Taken together, these components reinforced the widely adopted "triple aim" or "three-part aim" of better care for individuals, better health for populations, and reduction of per capita cost of healthcare.[29] The PCMH model was initially seen as a vehicle for achieving these goals in a practical way.

Healthcare systems in New York City like Mount Sinai began to implement the PCMH care model in earnest around the same time as they experimented with the ACO payment structure in 2012, and in combination, they represented a potentially new way to improve the value of healthcare that was being delivered, particularly primary care for elderly patients. Since Mount Sinai was developing its PCMH approach around the same time that City Health Works was launched, their respective leadership saw an opportunity for building bridges with the neighborhood while primary care was being redefined. City Health Works needed to find its own coach to navigate the swiftly changing context. There was no place more experienced with the PCMH model than Massachusetts, where even historically competitive healthcare systems across the state had formed unusually close relationships with each other to move forward together into uncharted territory.

Ever since 2006, when Massachusetts initiated healthcare reform under Governor Mitt Romney, the state has been ahead of the curve on a range of issues that other states will face, including states that have foregone ACA expansion. Back in 2006, Cambridge Health Alliance (CHA), a healthcare system with 11 percent of the state's mental health hospitalizations, was on the verge of financial collapse after rapid Medicaid expansion led the state to consider defunding the safety net. Its leadership, trying to envision what the situation would look like nine years ahead, in 2015, saw an opportunity. They thought that public healthcare within the context of universal access could achieve the triple aim of better health for individuals and populations at a lower cost. Recognizing that the 2006 financial model simply didn't support the kind of integrated, preventive, team-based primary care and behavioral health services that the population needed, CHA chose to proactively work with payers to flip its financial model from volume to value. It rapidly adopted the ACO model to restructure how it was paid and recognized that it needed equivalent changes in how primary and specialty care was delivered using the PCMH model. Along the way, they would need to build a new organizational culture, craft new partnerships with community organizations and neighborhood members, and create a high-functioning, proactive, population-oriented primary care model.

Fortunately, CHA was uniquely structured with a healthcare delivery system and a public health system under one roof and a strong and long history of supporting infrastructure for community health. Rather than simply fiddling with incentives and payments as means to toggle utilization and improve behaviors, the underlying workflows of healthcare personnel, patients, and neighborhood-based organizations was completely reassembled. CHA's pioneering approach, which embraced public health methods, community organizing, and local development efforts, was chronicled in case studies, scholarship, and elaborated in toolkits. [30] It was a good place to find a coach.

A HEALTHCARE SYSTEM COACH

In Revere, Massachusetts, a clinic site in the CHA network, Soma Stout began her work as a primary care physician where opiate addiction (e.g., oxycontin and heroin) was the leading cause of death among people under 65. Revere was home to one of the CHA sites, and Stout played an integral role in CHA's transformative journey as Vice President of PCMH Development in addition to being a physician. She was part of the CHA in 2008, when the sheer scale of financial threat to its existence required a completely new approach to healthcare system redesign: figure out what it would take for primary care teams to work in transformative ways with their patients and then determine how to pay for it. This meant that the quality of each connection with any and all staff at the CHA had to reinforce the patient's motivation to improve health.

By treating this as a cultural as well as a technical transformation, Stout began the PCMH journey for people all across CHA by having them take on the role of different patients. They had to reimagine what their healthcare system should look like from a first-person perspective that resonated with them. Importantly, patients were integrated into this process, including Cristin Lind, the young mother who took care of the little boy named Gabe whom we met earlier. She drew the now-famous diagram (figure 7.1) to help the team understand what her son needed to live a healthy life. In a process that Stout described as "meaning making," the groups of staff and patients began to organically name the components of the PCMH approach, extending their view to natural partners in the neighborhood as well as public health and social service organizations: "The idea of our health system functioning as 'a patient-centered medical neighborhood, functioning seamlessly as a practice without walls' emerged organically from this visioning process, creating enormous inspiration because it felt like a natural extension of our mission and core strengths as an organization."[31]

With examples of kids like Gabe, the CHA staff realized that any partnership that would benefit their patients was "within bounds" of a healthcare system. In the first year of the transformation, rather than obtaining advice from consultants, Stout invited over a hundred frontline staff (the majority of whom were from the community), midlevel leaders, and patients to propose how the transformation should be implemented over a six-month period. Senior leaders were invited to participate in these workgroups as well, ranging from care redesign to collaboration across departments to data and metrics to compensation, creating a grassroots to grasstops connected process.

Together they created a practical, achievable, and inspiring blueprint for transformation that drew from best practices outside but leveraged assets and implementation strategies inside to create a plan that was at once inspiring and deeply owned. Stout and a visionary organizational development leader, Marcy Lidman, simultaneously created an internal leadership academy to help a critical mass of midlevel leaders across the continuum (and across physician, nursing, and administrative leadership) develop capacity and confidence to lead to the transformation. By the end of the first year, a critical mass of "change" leaders emerged at every level of the organization who saw themselves as the champions of the vision; 94 percent of frontline receptionists and medical assistants could correctly identify the strategy, felt it was important to them, and understood that they had a critical role to play and knowledge and expertise from living in the community that mattered. A team of staff and patients were put into more formal "practice improvement teams" which to this day operate in every practice to continually improve health and care. As this process grew across the CHA system, the team framed problems and suggested solutions that were backed by data. But to move forward, they needed the financial resources to match. This is usually where many bottom-up initiatives stall, whether they emanate from the neighborhood or the healthcare system. In Stout's words, the intrinsic motivation that moves people to begin running toward a shared vision has to somehow transform into gliding before the will to run is exhausted. It's a hopeful vision, but even gliding, which sounds like a pipe dream for most healthcare systems, takes ongoing investment, extraordinary skill, and alignment with the winds of change.

As Stout recounts, CHA's CEO at the time, Dennis Keefe, had the courage to state that the organization needed to find out what was worth doing first, and then build a model of financing to follow. In their early adoption of the ACO and PCMH models, they were so far ahead of the nation that both concepts were literally being formed as they learned, and they leaned heavily on their staff and patients to navigate the way forward, instead of tasking an insular committee to define it for them. As a result, CHA survived the immediate financial threat, and a majority of their 100,000 primary care patients were paid for in the new modes of reimbursement, all while wait times for appointments reduced, cancer screening rates improved, hospitalizations for patients with diabetes dropped by 36 percent, and new healthcare and neighborhood partnerships flourished.[32] Peer-to-peer supports became integrated at every step of the system: the medical assistant serving as a health coach to her patients; a mental health care partner coaching someone to be resilient; suboxone treatment and support groups who helped each other to achieve breakthrough outcomes; or community health workers who helped people navigate through their health, social, and healthcare needs. To this day, proactive population management, health coaching, and frontline improvement is largely run by medical assistants and receptionists. They may not have advanced degrees, but they have deep relationships with their patients and systems to support them in a team environment in a way that transforms the health of patients and community. Recognizing the potential among these workers, CHA created scholarships and pathways for frontline staff to advance professionally, leading to a significant percentage of receptionists and medical assistants—who suddenly knew that they not only had the skills to answer phones but also the wisdom to be in relationship with their neighbors in a way that could transform lives—becoming the first people in their families to achieve a professional degree and emerge stably out of poverty.[33]

Stout isn't viewed as the *cause* of these improvements; rather, she harnessed the latent motivation and creativity of healthcare employees across CHA—from medical assistants to physicians to receptionists—who coached their more skeptical colleagues into seeing what they knew was possible. On a personal level, Stout is the type of person who immediately melts the personal and professional divide with her enveloping hugs. She moves with the energy of a community organizer and the lightness of a former dancer, rapidly shifting attention away from herself to the groups that she is perpetually assembling. Her background is hard to place; her childhood in densely populated Calcutta, India, and elite education at Harvard College, UCSF medical school, Brigham and Women's, and Boston Children's Hospital seem to cancel each other out as she maintains a firm anchor in the present moment. Where some doctors who have rapidly scaled the hierarchal medical establishment wear their accomplishments as a chip on their shoulder, Stout is hurtling forward on a journey that she feels has only just begun; whereas most healthcare system transformation[34] leaders come from highly disciplined backgrounds of financing, information technology, quality improvement, or specialty care, she speaks from experience about the journey of moving "healthcare to focus upon health" with a tidal wave of enthusiasm; while the health economists of her generation were busy drafting conceptual frameworks that would form the bulwark of the ACA, Stout was learning what healthcare had to do with the more intuitive goal of living a healthier life, in the broadest sense. At some point in her training at UCSF and the Harvard hospitals between 1993 and 2003, she would undoubtedly have rubbed shoulders with elite leaders who shape and define the healthcare sector as we know it. However, she deliberately sought insights in places off-center from the self-reverential locales in which she had trained. While at UC-Berkeley UCSF, she immersed herself in the rural countryside of Guyana to understand how an entire district can take an integrated view on their own development that included education, economics, and social inclusion. In Boston, her career took off in the suburbs. Along the way, she didn't squeeze efficiences out of existing systems to "bend the cost curve," the mantra of her economist colleagues: instead she created an entirely new playbook.

Being part of an environment where coaching culture is valued makes an uncertain journey more likely to succeed. Because the right path forward for CHA was not specified in model descriptions or standards, Stout and her colleagues found ways to engage people on the journey through peer learning systems called learning collaboratives.

To help each other in the broader context of Massachusetts's healthcare reform, for example, CHA joined other Harvard-affiliated hospitals in an Academic Innovations Collaborative (AIC), which is part of an effort across 20 Harvard-affiliated primary care teaching practices to create an environment where members can coach one another on the problems they encounter and solutions they discover. As I sat in on an AIC gathering in April 2014, the process that I saw Stout facilitating seemed very similar to the MI approach that City Health Works coaches use to interact with their clients. There was one major difference, however. As a group facilitator, she redirects individual issues back toward the group so they can share their insight. For example, when a member of the group who worked at one institution shared that her hospital may not support the AIC, Stout could hear her disappointment and diminished motivation:

> *Stout*: I can imagine that this news is incredibly demoralizing.
> *Comment*: [*nods*] Budget issues, as usual. Across the board. If primary care comes up with funding on its own, then they can do what they like.
> *Stout*: It's a different message that we're not committed to primary care versus there is a lot going on at this time and we can't commit to it all at this time.
> [*she pauses, redirects to the group*]

When you're on a hang glider there is all that energy when you're running and getting ready to launch. This two years has been about going
from static to moving. So one of the big picture issues is financial sustainability. When you're getting from running to gliding, how do you
think about the new activities in the gliding phase? Otherwise you keep
running, and you don't have the resources and energies to keep running.
What do you think it takes to be successful to make that kind of shift?[35]

As I listened to Stout speak, I heard a system-level coach at work using
a different set of operating principles than what traditional medical education offers. By directly confronting the tension that an individual issue
represented, she was able to engage a larger group in an adaptive problem-
solving exercise that generated many ways to approach a challenge. In her
discussions at CHA or in a larger group format of motivated individuals, she
remained focused on how healthcare systems *enable* patients to assemble
healthier lives, rather than adding stress and friction to their effort. This
allows people who work in healthcare to bring their experience to bear in
solving problems in concert with their technical expertise. When healthcare
professionals operate along these lines, they begin to see the neighborhood
and its people as their partners in health, rather than simply their current
and future patients. Rather than being somewhere in the middle of a clinical hierarchy, a truly patient-centric approach flattens power dynamics that
lead to dangerous dependence on strategies that lead to consistently poor
results. Instead of asking why the insight of a health coach like Melendez or
Cruz should influence how primary care is designed and delivered, the right
question is how the healthcare system can shift its center of gravity toward
the neighborhood, where people live. Whoever can contribute should be
part of an improvement-oriented discussion.

Even with all of these operating principles working in concert, questions
of economics and financing loom. Although the ACO and PCMH models are
incremental opportunities for healthcare systems to make a shift outside of
hospitals, they represent relatively small opportunities in the broader financial portfolio of healthcare systems. As the deputy director of the Center of
Medicaid and Medicare Innovations Center, Rahul Rajkumar, states, "How
we pay for health at scale matters."[36]

8

The Center Cannot Hold

The central idea underlying all these efforts is this: to accelerate the pace of change, we must take different, reinforcing actions simultaneously in a concerted effort to turn a behemoth health care complex into a more streamlined health system . . . we must tackle the problem in its entirety and on all fronts.

—Dr. Harvey Fineberg, former president of the Institute of Medicine

CHANGE IS CONSTANT

In a personal conversation I had with a healthcare management consultant, I learned that roughly 1 trillion of nearly 3 trillion healthcare sector dollars is expected to move from old institutions to new actors and intermediaries in the next decade. In fact, this particular management consulting company was being asked to facilitate the creation of a city-level "health platform" where healthcare systems, private sector companies, and the "local community" could work together to achieve long-term health goals. This dynamism at the sector level is triggered by large-scale federal and state-led reform and sustained by market dynamics that create opportunities to displace inefficient and complacent healthcare architecture in favor of systems shaped by the needs of end users. According to Joy Johnson Wilson, who has been with the National Council of State Legislators since 1978 and now serves as director of Health and Human Services Policy, our healthcare at the state and local level is undergoing a degree of dynamism that is difficult to keep up with: "It's like cars going by really fast. I've never seen a time like it. There is excitement and terror."[1] These dynamics allow for a promising horizon, but the question remains: how can all the pieces of the puzzle be brought together to enable a true shift toward neighborhood-centric healthcare?

For the time being, the financial incentives to make this shift are ill defined and uncertain. Experts like Soma Stout are working to build the healthcare systems of the future even as their organizations continue to struggle. Judging by financials alone, it is evident that the Cambridge Health Alliance, including Stout's Patient Centered Medical Home (PCMH) initiatives, has had to carefully monitor revenues to preserve the viability of the safety-net system. In 2011, 85 percent of CHA's net patient revenue came from two of its hospitals, whereas the nonhospital realm where Stout's work resides, which is largely clinic-based, accounted for merely 15 percent.[2] At the same time, the effectiveness of clinic and community-based services actively threatens the solvency of CHA hospitals despite a spate of alternative payment models to reduce the powerful financial logic of keeping heads in beds. From Stout's perspective, the system had to ensure that it was rapidly providing new primary care growth to balance the decrease in hospitalizations. It also had to find ways to keep patients at the far-lower-cost, high-quality CHA hospitals, rather than having them go to more expensive brand-named Boston hospitals for common medical conditions. Fortunately, during this time CHA grew from 75,000 to 100,000 patients, allowing this financially precarious transformation in healthcare delivery to proceed, albeit carefully.

By taking activities out of the hospital and into a primary care setting, and even a step further by helping people assemble healthier lives in their neighborhoods with minimal clinical support, Stout effectively set the wheels in motion to bankrupt the trio of hospitals supporting CHA's network. Partners Healthcare lost $22 million from its bottom line in 2014 because of its acquisition of the Neighborhood Health Plan, which largely covers patients just like Delta and Ray.[3] Compared to the 6 cents on the dollar that Mount Sinai Hospital was losing on patients like Ray in 2011, Partners lost 20 cents. How healthcare is paid for and how changes in payment support more effective care models remain central concerns for state-based and nationwide reform efforts.

The battle to demonstrate financial value is not unique to CHA. In Pennsylvania, for example, a group of practices and healthcare insurance plans implemented a PCMH model as part of the Southeastern Pennsylvania Chronic Care Initiative. Their effort was studied by a team of academics at Brigham and Women's Hospital, the University of Pennsylvania, and the RAND Corporation. The results were, to put it nicely, incremental: the effort

"was associated with limited improvements in quality and was not associated with reductions in utilization of hospital, emergency department, or
ambulatory care services or total costs over 3 years."[4] Obviously, administrators looking for a quick fix are not going to find it in reform undertakings
of this kind. Back in Texas, Fred Cerise announced that none of Parkland's
57 vice presidents would receive bonus pay because of the public system's
weak financial performance in 2014—a decision that was unanimously
supported by their board.[5]

And yet, in every single setting, the transformation of healthcare systems,
including large-scale experimentation with unprecedented neighborhood-
based architecture, is accelerating. In response to the independent study
about the Pennsylvania group's results, its participants forcefully responded
that their effort was worth it:

> Collaboration between primary care physicians and payers now provides a
> platform for data sharing and collaborative care management efforts that
> may lead to additional improvements in quality and patient experience,
> and reduction in waste. The state has demonstrated how its leadership
> and facilitation can bring together stakeholders for valuable collaboration.
> New training programs are teaching young primary care practitioners and
> inter-professional teams learn new ways of delivering care [sic]. Physicians,
> medical groups, health systems, insurers and the state have found common
> ground.[6]

The cost of this transformative process does not adequately capture its
value, but both cost and value are independent of the participants' overwhelming belief that it was worth doing. Another way to look at these financial losses is that they are investments into our nation's future healthcare
system architecture, borne at the organizational level. There are public
sector–led and market-driven forces at work that add momentum to this
process of change, giving rise to a new generation of ethical change agents,
like Cerise, Stout, Doran Schrantz, and Donya Williams: they all play an integral role in distributing authority within their organizations, and interde-
pendently with other organizations, so the ensemble can effectively search
for a way forward. As Cerise's professional path demonstrates, even being
publically fired by Louisiana's governor did not slow his transition to a new
setting that embraced his principled leadership. In Texas, where marquee

components of federal healthcare reform continue to be rejected, efforts to build new healthcare system architecture continue unabated.

BUILDING MOMENTUM

The cadence of change in healthcare architecture is quickening as a host of new efforts drive a shift from healthcare systems toward neighborhoods. National desire for improved quality and value in healthcare is translating into myriad local efforts. In 2012 the Centers for Medicare and Medicaid Services Innovation Center funded more than two dozen projects to assess community health workers' impact and cost. Academics have taken notice, and the Penn Center for Community Health Workers, NYU's Department of Population Health, and others are trying to resolve practical tension between their potential benefit to healthcare systems (a source of financing) and their primary service to cultural communities and local neighborhoods.[7] For-profit companies have experimented with ways to offer services within communities as well. Integra Services Connect built a multistate community health worker model ("feet-on-the-street"), which is used in places including New York City and Hennepin County, Minnesota.[8] The venture-capital-backed Iora Health integrates health coaches into their primary care model. At the same time, technology companies like Omada Health have successfully scaled up online coaches who virtually support people in their homes across the country. Manatt Health, a private consulting company, teamed up with Commonwealth Fund, a respected healthcare policy group, to clarify the business case for organizations like City Health Works and Health Leads.[9] Policy-focused bodies, like the Institute of Medicine and California Health Workforce Alliance, have focused on how to "mainstream" their presence[10] and sharpen their role,[11] respectively. As Dave Chokshi and I wrote in the *New England Journal of Medicine*, rising domestic attention to community health workers has inspired interest in global settings with more experience with the practical challenges domestic initiatives are only beginning to encounter.[12]

In order to move a dense cloud of national activity into a regional or local setting, there need to be clear ways to facilitate the adoption of proven and promising solutions like community health workers, who have an integral role but uncertain place in the constellation of healthcare systems, public health activities, and neighborhood development. This will require redesigning organizational and financial structures so that these models can operate as a fundamental part of our health system, rather than being seen as an add-on.

RETHINKING MEDICAID

As the implications of national healthcare reform were being felt at the local and regional level by healthcare systems, mostly through the federally administered Medicare program, many states saw opportunities to redesign their Medicaid operations. All states believed that if they had more latitude to shift away from largely healthcare facility–centric models it would be possible to manage Medicaid at lower cost *and* improved outcomes. But because there was no national blueprint for how the unique confluence of payment reform, healthcare delivery redesign, and local considerations should be reliably constructed, accomplishing this required learning by doing, through CMS-supported programs like the State Innovation Models (SIM).[13] Permission to modify a state's Medicaid program is given in the form of a "waiver," allowing the state to experiment outside the standard rules. The opportunity to redesign Medicaid even enticed states like Indiana, which had originally rejected expansion of Medicaid with federal subsidies, on the condition that it could make it more consumer driven.[14] This was not a quid pro quo arrangement for accepting federal support; states like Texas, which continue to reject the expansion of their state Medicaid program with federal subsidies, have still been granted waivers to redesign their existing Medicaid program.[15] For states like New York that had embraced not only the Medicaid expansion but also the full breadth of programs such as ACOs, redesign of Medicaid and Medicare could theoretically take place in tandem.

Massachusetts, which has led the nation in nearly all aspects of healthcare reform, again pointed the way by creating a waiver that parlayed $628 million into incentive payments in seven safety-net healthcare systems based upon performance improvements between 2012 and 2014. CHA was one of these healthcare systems.[16] The statewide effort was called the Delivery System Transformation Initiative (DSTI), and it is no coincidence that its goals align with what CHA was already doing. All areas of performance improvement within DSTI were focused upon preparing safety-net healthcare systems to better assess if a patient should be taken care of in a hospital, where costs were highest and overtreatment posed substantial risks to patient health, versus in a clinic or the neighborhood. The four areas where performance would be measured were designed to encourage innovation in how care is conceived, delivered, paid for, and measured:

- Development of a fully integrated delivery system built on Patient-Centered Medical Home principles;
- Implementation of innovative care models to improve quality of care and health outcomes;
- Development of capabilities necessary to implement alternative payment models;
- Population-focused health outcome improvements.[17]

In some ways, CHA benefited from being in dire financial straits. They were able to work with the state and other safety-net healthcare systems to create the aforementioned waiver that redesigned how they were paid.[18] By participating, CHA became part of a coalition of healthcare systems that formed a nascent "learning system."[19] Although the idea of learning across healthcare systems has percolated for years, the work of cooperating and exchanging approaches with potential competitors was new to most participants, especially to executives (the "C-Suite") of hospitals and healthcare systems. Today, a larger learning system has formed across Massachusetts, many years into the state's healthcare reform process. As the four areas for performance improvement indicate, the DSTI does not prescribe how exactly its aims translate into organization-level activities. Instead, healthcare systems like CHA found regional partners to learn with, like Lawrence General Hospital, where I visited with Stout at a DSTI meeting of hospital executives who had come together to discuss how to better link resources devoted to reducing readmissions to related efforts. In fact, a representative from PCCI was on hand to share their experience at Parkland.

In 2014, New York State unfurled a $6.4 billion Delivery System Reform Incentive Payment (DSRIP), to "fundamentally restructure the health care delivery system."[20] Compared to DSTI, DSRIP involves many more actors, more money, and therefore more complexity. It also has more prescribed organizational-level goals. The top-level DSRIP goal is clearly stated: "reduce avoidable hospital use by 25 percent over 5 years." Equally important, the state initially resolved not to increase the Medicaid budget even as more people were projected to be on Medicaid. Simultaneously they were moving from volume to value-based payments. In a state where the healthcare systems are so large that they can exert effective counter political pressure on the state, New York State agreed to give participating healthcare systems a one-time injection of *conditional* financing between 2015 and 2020. The condition was that it would be performance-based and would be predicated upon how effectively healthcare systems formally incorporated hundreds of service agencies and neighborhood partners into delivering care to Medicaid patients.

Healthcare systems that chose to participate—like Mount Sinai Healthcare System and the Health and Hospital Corporation (HHC)—stand alongside large organized groups of physicians called Independent Practice Associations (IPAs) and are called Performing Provider Systems (PPSs). Each PPS has an overlapping set of partners that link them to each other in a complex network of organizational relationships that is simultaneously tangled and reflective of how their patients move around the city to access care. Unlike PCCI's step-by-step, deliberate efforts to bring Dallas neighborhood organizations like the Bridge to co-design their relationship, or Hennepin's deliberate development of county-level healthcare and public health systems, New York DSRIP put hundreds of organizations together—including competing and conflicting ones—to build their collective destiny under the pressure of time, performance, and payments. It was the everything-all-at-once approach I had seen in integrated development projects abroad, which definitely shifted the center of gravity to the neighborhood, but it lacked clear guidance on how to make sense of a new context. Everyone would have to figure it out together, or fail together.

For Harlem Hospital or Elmhurst Hospital, which are both part of HHC, the decision to participate was obvious, since they care predominantly for low-income New Yorkers, who are covered by state Medicaid. Hybrid systems like the Mount Sinai Health System had a different incentive to participate. According to CEO Ken Davis, the sheer scale of people served through the DSRIP process would enable the system to invest in an adaptive neighborhood strategy that could cushion it from ambiguity in the inevitable tweaking and recalibration of federal Medicare and Medicaid payments. "To mitigate that risk," Davis asserts, "hospitals need to broaden the populations they serve, and offer services that cover a larger geographical area. ... The larger net also allows hospitals to learn from different patient populations, such as the elderly, and make strategic decisions to improve their care."[21] Since Mount Sinai had become a much larger health system after its merger, it assumed the care of many more Medicaid patients and is formally designated a safety-net system along with HHC. However, it receives healthcare payments from both public and private insurance arrangements, yet cannot build two fundamentally separate healthcare systems. In the best case, this means that populations who have private insurance will also experience more neighborhood-centric care, while Medicaid and Medicare patients will benefit from investments driven by private insurers like telemedicine services and higher-quality patient experience.

Each participating PPS is required to be part of a larger network of social agencies and neighborhood-based organizations that it must pay, also on a performance basis, to improve outcomes, lower costs, and reduce hospitalizations. The "arranged marriage" of the social sector and healthcare systems comes with the need for considerable adjustment when accounting for different expectations, modes of operating, and ways of exchanging mission-critical information. This could amount to a direct transfer of healthcare sector finances to an increasingly squeezed social sector. However, the details of execution matter immensely, particularly in an environment where most social sector organizations and agencies are decades behind equivalent investments in information technology, financial systems, and methods of demonstrating accountability. Although the DSRIP process has months of planning time built in, the sums of money sound astronomical to beleaguered community-based organizations and social service agencies, whereas health systems are still gauging how much to incorporate the DSRIP process into their core population health strategies. The absence of "cheap talk" between these distant sectors prior to this process almost guarantees that the solutions that emerge will be crude at best without the participation of intermediaries like community development financing institutions (CDFIs), who have the expertise to structure the investment interface between neighborhood organizations and healthcare systems.[22]

New York's DSRIP includes four domains of redesign: (1) overall progress and effectiveness of redesign; (2) system transformation; (3) clinical improvement; and (4) populationwide improvement. Examining the dense logic models and publicly available Gantt charts that describe how a healthcare system will achieve even one goal in a domain, it is clear that the effort underway has all the engineering complexity of building a new bridge. Ironically, the entire point of the DSRIP is to connect New York State healthcare systems to their own neighborhoods so people do not get lost in an ocean of complexity that inevitably takes a toll on their health. Five nearby health-care systems in the New York City area—NYU, Montefiore, Northshore-LIJ, HHC, and New York–Presbyterian—each have a different strategic outlook on the DSRIP process that reflects their competitive position.[23] At a high level, all embrace their newfound roles of stewards of health in the neighborhood, yet their respective business strategies represent distinctive interpretations of what infrastructure they will build to fulfill this aim. In the grand tradition of New York State public works, like the immense clusters of public housing projects, it will behoove the co-architects of DSRIP to remember that New Yorkers aim to stay in their neighborhoods, not in healthcare systems, to live healthier lives.

REDEFINING THE "H"

In New York and beyond, pioneers from a multitude of backgrounds have been working on innovative ways to rework old systems to better meet the needs of both patients and budget-constrained health systems. For example, the work of "connecting settings" has been traditionally accomplished in a simple but costly manner: 911 system + ambulance. Over the past few years, pioneers in emergency medicine like Mount Sinai's Kevin Munjal have been rethinking the role of emergency medical technicians (EMTs) as initiating basic care in homes instead of reflexively bringing everybody to the hospital.[24] The Office of the National Coordinator (ONC) is shepherding literally hundreds of technology startups to "connect settings" through apps.[25] On the West Coast, Oregon State's coordinated care organizations, which cover specific geographic service areas, have not only invested in community health workers, but have also brought residents into the planning process for targeting Medicaid funds.[26] Even the historic tradition of home visits by clinicians is making a comeback. The Visiting Doctors Program at Mount Sinai, founded by socially minded residents in 1993, has been previously supported by philanthropy; now connections like these form the basis for a "structural redesign of healthcare" and are being recognized within Mount Sinai Health System and nationally for their anticipated benefit.[27] Two of the three resident co-founders of the Visiting Doctors Program are now systemwide leaders: David Muller is dean of Medical Education and Jeremy Boal is the chief medical officer, both with substantial influence across the city's largest healthcare system. Over at HHC, two relatively young practitioners and scholars of population health who met in medical school at the University of Pennsylvania and trained together at Brigham and Women's Hospital, Dave Chokshi and Nicholas Stine, have earned senior positions that defy the usual hierarchy of the medical establishment.

Much of this work falls under the catchall umbrella of population health management, which has propelled a new generation of private companies like Evolent Health to their stratospheric $1 billion valuation in anticipation of a major shift away from hospitals toward neighborhood-centric and community-organized care. It is a nationwide trend that is echoed by the American Hospital Association (AHA):

> Hospitals and health care systems in the United States are focused on redefining the "H"—that is, exploring what it means to be a hospital in a rapidly transforming health care environment....To meet these challenges, hospitals and health care system leaders will need to lead the way in forging community collaborations that:
> - Appropriately allocate resources and define a shared responsibility for improving community health
> - Bring insight, perspective and support from the community into the hospital board room as hospital leaders consider paths for transformation
> - Enter into strategic partnerships for improving community health and health outcomes.[28]

Of course, the practice of meaningfully integrating the hundreds of neighborhood, community, and faith-based organizations as well as larger, citywide social services, into healthcare system processes is abstract and fraught with concern on all sides. With hundreds of millions of dollars at stake, the choice of investing into systems like PCCI in Dallas versus social movement platforms like ISAIAH in Minneapolis–St. Paul depends upon who is making the decision. Instead of choosing one or the other, both are likely necessary, which presents fundamental design challenges for how healthcare systems incorporate them. Even if an optimal combination were possible, what would this mean in practice for New York City's people and neighborhoods? Who will arbitrate when they inevitably veer off course, favoring technology over social mobilization, or vice versa?

THE ROLE OF INTEGRATORS

To substantively improve health in the neighborhood and its populations, healthcare systems, public health organizations, and social movements must identify and invest in working through "local integrators."[29] This is no easy task since there is no strict formula for what a local integrator looks like or how many may exist in a neighborhood. However, there are some common features: an integrator is (1) trusted by other local organizations (including other integrators) to facilitate agreements about shared long-term goals and committed to help track progress; (2) continuously learning from and integrating information from traditional silos (e.g., education, social services, job training, healthcare) to ensure that individuals appreciate direct benefits from "population health" improvements;[30] and (3) working at the systems level to connect other integrators, spreading information about approaches that work, and planning for the sustainability of collective effort.[31]

It is no surprise that a "local integrator" sounds like the elusive unicorn. In practice, this is a role filled by many organizations, ranging from public agencies like the New York City Department of Health to New York City's neighborhood development thought leaders like Anthony Bugg-Levine of the NonProfit Finance Fund (a CDFI), who developed the field of impact investing, to Rosanne Haggerty of Community Solutions, a "MacArthur Genius" who developed the nationally successful 100,000 Homes campaign to mobilize neighborhoods to reduce homelessness, to Ben Hecht of Living Cities, who fuses investment strategies with practical opportunities that span urban and suburban boundaries. The common thread is a commitment to shared responsibility and citizenship for the health of a people within a geographic place.

In recognition of the need for local integrators in New York, City Health Works has been asked to co-lead multiple work streams within DSRIP by the Mount Sinai Health System.[32] As Manmeet Kaur carefully navigates requests from insurance companies, healthcare systems, and technology companies who recognize City Health Works's role as a bridge to the neighborhood, she also keeps her sights set on a sustainable business model to invest in her staff and organization. Fortunately, philanthropic funders like the Robert Wood Johnson Foundation and the Robin Hood Foundation have recognized that the process of building a health system with the neighborhood at its center requires research and development to overcome the short-term pressures of nonprofit philanthropy and revenue targets. Their ongoing support helps balance out the traditional target objectives (e.g. HEDIS scores [the Healthcare Effectiveness Data and Information Set] or managed Medicaid and Medicare star-ratings) stipulated by healthcare systems like Mount Sinai, which has contracted with City Health Works to provide a service to low-income and elderly patients. For now, the greatest pressures come from where they should: in the form of the Wednesday morning meetings where the hive of activity led by City Health Works coaches concentrates insights to help the organization evolve.

As Columbia sociologist David Stark puts it, "entrepreneurship is the ability to keep multiple orders of worth in play and to exploit the resulting ambiguity."[33] When individuals with diverse perspectives in an organization are able to respond to different and competing aims, they find ways to move forward that reduce ambiguity even as change remains constant. Organizations and individuals that play the role of integrators constantly encounter possible avenues of divergent action that must be carefully calibrated with their capabilities. They are expert at finding satisfactory and sufficient solutions to complex problems, which honors the notion that in the long run, they have a diversity of experiences and develop a robust set of skills that become particularly crucial in moments of transformation. Where others see crisis, they see opportunities to restore balance. In my view, this quest is best organized in the neighborhood, but connected across the country, where a diverse array of individuals, organizations, and social networks can collaborate in fulfilling our street-level healthcare promise.

ESCAPE VELOCITY

Not every neighborhood in the country needs to develop expertise in all aspects of health improvement—that's the beauty of the integrator concept. On the other hand, with lots of individual hives of activity swirling about simultaneously across the country, with increasingly innovative collaborative technology to match, the opportunity for highly tailored channels of information sharing is too promising to pass up. As the public health sector catches up with modern technology, is it possible to imagine an interwoven network of information-sharing hubs that trade expertise in improving veteran health, for example, or support early childhood development in very concrete ways? What if there was so much coordinated energy pulsing across the country that groups like City Health Works could easily see their own role in the neighborhood more clearly, instead of simply grasping for it?

In some ways, these networks are already forming. At the local level, Single Stop USA specifically focuses on integrating a neighborhood's safety-net services and plans to expand beyond its 113 locations across 8 states according to its public plan. At the neighborhood level, organizations like Communities Joined in Action have formed large-scale learning networks of more than 150 places that share toolkits and peer mentorship in online platforms and physical meetings. Groups like Health Leads are natural aggregators that enable patients to build a healthier life by providing anything from legal services to nutritious food. For more problem-solving-oriented networks, Community Solutions used a campaign format to create a network of 186 places across the country to find homes for 105,000 homeless Americans, while the National Institute for Children's Health Quality has used a "collaborative innovation network" structure to reduce infant mortality in ways that draw upon the collective intelligence of experts. The Network for Regional Healthcare Improvement works to bridge national and state payment reform initiatives with regional problem-solving networks. A group of 40 of the nation's leading healthcare systems formed a network called the Institute for Health Improvement Leadership Alliance to complement these neighborhood and expert networks with a strategy to drive "change from the inside out" of healthcare. There are dozens of other learning networks, each trying to provide a piece of the broader puzzle that can improve health in the neighborhood. So many, in fact, that it can be hard for a neighborhood or healthcare system to know how to get the most relevant and pertinent insights amid a thicket of learning collaboratives.

Stout often speaks about "ah-ha!" moments in the journey of clinical transformation. These moments allow participants to break out of patterns of traditional decision-making as they see a more promising pathway emerge. She found that having patients present when CHA was making strategic decisions was deeply motivating for nonclinical staff, who in turn created the momentum for clinical staff to see their shifting responsibilities in a new light. Once her clinic was organized into motivated teams, she recognized that she would need to have hard conversations with her organization's leadership about financing. Because everyone on the frontline was ready and participated in the visioning process, the comprehensive change that Stout proposed was an easier sell to her leadership and board. In retrospect, hers seems like a smooth story, one without false starts, unproductive eddies, and moments of frustration. Of course, that is not how anything hard really is, and along the way, Stout recognized that participants at all levels had experienced moments of hard-earned insight that could be shared with others on a similar journey. She calls the trail of transformation "glide paths" and she believed they could be communicated across the nation.

Stout's vision for this kind of national information sharing put her in contact with a communications and strategy expert who understood population health from many perspectives: Gail Freeman, former vice president of strategy and chief marketing officer at the Institute for Healthcare Improvement, the organization where the "triple aim" was coined. Freeman and Stout began discussing how difficult it was to move beyond the orbit of business as usual in healthcare, even when an entire organization or learning collaborative was trying mightily to do so. Both of them, they discovered, were admirers of the work of Jim Hester, an aerospace engineer and social scientist who has played a significant role in rationalizing how Vermont's healthcare sector serves its people. His specialty resides in systems architecting, an engineering discipline that stresses the social elements of building something that is hard to imagine, moving "from a vague concept and limited resources to a satisfactory and feasible system concept and executable program."[34] To express the spirit behind this concept, Hester often starts his talks with an inspirational story about how the Apollo mission to the moon was conceived, starting with the goals, values, and aims that motivated a *successful* moonshot. Inspired by Hester's career, Stout and Freeman used the metaphor of achieving escape velocity to a distant goal. "Escape Velocity: 100 Million Healthier Lives (100M)" was born.

As Stout worked on formulating central tenets of this initiative, she started thinking about those "ah-ha" moments that had shaped her experience at Cambridge Health Alliance—moments that were taking place ad infinitum across the country, across different places, healthcare systems, and organizations that saw themselves as being integral to health improvement. All of the pioneers I encountered were working with a limited set of partners to grapple with the challenges of making an unwieldy sector work as advertised. Instead of simply capturing the work of pioneers as case studies or research monographs, the 100M team wanted to harness the glide paths and facilitate their immediate application by other parts of a growing network. These proof points, or "bright spots," as the 100M team began calling them, contained the big and little excursions that healthcare systems, neighborhoods, and caregivers like Cristin Lind were taking to build healthier lives at different scales, from many to one. The basic premise was that what was needed to advance the yet-hazy goal of "100 million healthier lives" was not one specific action or set of activities to be planned, executed, and measured, but rather the development of a new set of continuously learning networks.

This point cannot be emphasized enough. 100M is not an advocacy campaign. It does not have a written set of policy proposals. It does not claim to have "the right answer" to improve health in the United States—nor does it claim that there *is* a single "right answer." What the group is trying to do instead is provide a platform for raising the right questions, and the movement to power it.

In many ways, 100M fits within two well-established themes in health policy. The first is a focus on "place-based" initiatives, which resurge to national prominence nearly every decade. In fact, a leader within the Escape Velocity initiative, Tyler Norris, helped to shape and lead the Healthy Communities Movement, which was the American offshoot of the WHO's Healthy Cities initiative back in 1989. The basic goal of all these movements was to translate decades of scattered expertise, insights, and experience into street-level improvement. A closely related aim is to shift away from large-scale, big-push regulatory reforms like the ACA. Earlier that year, Esther Dyson, a well-known technology venture capitalist who invests in healthcare companies, staged a competition for towns/cities to become one of five places on the "Way to Wellville." The winning Wellville participants were small towns in Oregon, Michigan, California, New York, and South Carolina. The Robert Wood Johnson Foundation, meanwhile, identified 20 places to work with in developing measures of a "culture of health," while other philanthropic efforts through groups like the Kresge, Kellogg, and California Endowment focused on locally driven improvement.

But again and again, these place-based initiatives have failed to produce sustained, continuous improvement on a large scale. That is because they focus on supporting a type of content—local policies on healthcare—rather than on creating a learning environment: one that sustains both the motivation and the ability to improve. That environment is what 100M is building. The campaign, which is hosted by the Institute of Healthcare

Improvement, serves as a "backbone" organization that coordinates activities of thematic hubs, channels financing, and provides technology and measurement support as needed across the country.

The concept of creating learning environments instead of content is not unique to 100M. Consider education: we don't hand five-year-old children the *Encyclopædia Britannica* and say, "see you in 12 years." Instead, we build schools that bring lots of kids together to discuss, ask questions, and explore. We provide them with tools for continuous discovery, from the Socratic method to the tenets of scientific inquiry. We provide guides and mentors in the form of teachers. Perhaps most importantly, in building the school and providing the tools and the teachers, we implicitly provide a motivating belief in the possibility of success: that if you do the work, and use the tools, and work with your teachers, you can keep getting better. Structures, tools, teachers, and motivation are precisely what 100M brings to the mission to improve health.

In more technical language, 100M is designing an interaction ecosystem for all of these individuals and organizations to sustain their relationships. Through those relationships, members can actively search for solutions within the network, draw expertise and experience into their neighborhoods, and share stories of success that motivate the journey. The echoes of 1:1 interaction, MI interviewing, and organizational methods used by Cambridge Health Alliance, ISAIAH, City Health Works, and the Dallas Information Exchange Portal are no accident: Stout and Freeman were aware of these dynamic data and information channels when they put together the Escape Velocity Conference. Their goal with 100M is to create a dynamic channel—actually, a network of channels—that can easily scale up to the level of the Centers for Medicare and Medicaid Innovations Center and down to the level of face to face. The nationally distributed leadership of the 100M Campaign aims to formalize a national search for new healthcare system designs that include our nation's neighborhoods, but also to build an exchange network for the inevitable diversity that emerges. 100M will be, at its finest, a multidimensional, high-tech, scalable glide path of national collaboration that will shift the center of healthcare into the neighborhood.

Where to begin? In her own version of a barn raising, Stout and her team began calling people and inviting them to the Escape Velocity event, where together they would launch the 100M Campaign. If the vision was too fuzzy, they created working groups to make it clear enough, which in turn drew individuals, organizations, and networks in to shape the event. When colleagues helpfully offered ideas for providing more specified content, like defining the metrics for the campaign up front, Stout gently but firmly resisted. Instead, her team listened intently to what people across the nation—from healthcare, public health, community development, and neighborhood— saw as necessary ingredients for the campaign to be successful. As the event drew closer, the call to attend felt more like an invitation to Woodstock than a technical conference. Excitement was generated by the sheer potential of bringing together nearly 200 people from almost 140 organizations across the country—ranging from Kaiser Permanente to the Veterans Administration to a rural town in western Oregon—who felt they had something to contribute. To attend, organizations pledged to submit action plans for what they could contribute to the campaign's goals. At the event, Stout's team promised to organize and share their collective assets, anything from money to serving as a regional or topical organizing hub. Finally, on October 8, 2014, at 2:52 PM, the entire Escape Velocity group committed to leading a movement that will result in 100 million healthier lives.

PART III

9

From Organizations to Integrators

I think there is a phenomenally deep connection between networks and goodness. I think the reason we form social networks in our lives is precisely to create and sustain all kinds of good and desirable properties.
—Nicholas Christakis

PIECES OF THE PUZZLE

A few months before the October 2014 Escape Velocity event in Boston, where the 100M Healthier Lives Campaign was launched, CNN led a series of investigations into grossly delayed care at the Veterans Affairs (VA) hospitals.[1] Many veterans died while waiting for treatment. The response to the exposé was swift: an internal Department of Veterans Affairs audit; an FBI investigation; a White House investigation; congressional hearings; resignations of top officials; recognition of a "corrosive culture" leading to "chronic and significant system failures."[2] The mix of a massive healthcare system, sluggish bureaucracy, and two powerfully hierarchal cultures—the military and medicine—was insular and deadly, despite successful quality improvement efforts in the past.[3] West Point graduate and former CEO of Procter and Gamble Robert McDonald became the 8th secretary of veterans affairs, replacing the respected 4-star general and 34th chief of staff of the army, Eric Shinseki, as the head of the Veterans Health Administration (VHA). This system of 1,700 sites of care serves nearly 9 million veterans each year. Secretary McDonald teamed up with Carolyn Clancy, former director of the Agency for Healthcare Research and Quality, to lead the organization through a rocky period of systemically changing its behavior amidst extraordinary public scrutiny.

The effects of the scandal echoed beyond the VHA. In May 2015, the Centers for Medicare and Medicaid Services hosted an event inspired by the 100M Campaign at their headquarters in Baltimore. The event, entitled the 100 Million Healthier Lives Summit, was remarkable because it brought together people from multiple federal agencies (e.g., U.S. Department of Agriculture and the Department of Defense), and their labyrinthine sub-programs, to understand how their efforts to improve the health of their respective constituents were related. Regan Crump, a former nurse and currently VHA's director of the Office of Strategic Planning and Analysis, stood at the front of the packed room and asked attendees to "stand up if you are active duty military or have served in the United States military!" About a dozen people stood up in a room of 60, including men and women in uniform. Crump continued, "now stand up if you're from a group outside of the VA that currently serves our nation's veterans." A dozen more stood up. He paused, "now stand up and come forward to give your name to my colleague if you'd like to connect what you're working on to improve the health of 20 million veterans." He quickly added, "the men and women in this room who have served this country are watching you!"

As I stood waiting to speak with Crump's colleague, I met a few other people working on veterans health in New York City who either represented organizations or themselves. As Crump announced the participation of his department in the 100M Healthier Lives Campaign, he provided some context for their enthusiasm: the past year's scandal had led his institution to look for more ways to serve as an active hub of support—a national integrator for veterans health across hundreds of local and national organizations—instead of behaving like a silo for healthcare service delivery.

Meanwhile, Soma Stout and her colleagues from the Institute for Healthcare Improvement (IHI) were readying the room for a more interactive and lively "mixer" to ensure that the main purpose of the day—building meaningful relationships between federal agency and nonfederal change agents—would have enough time to take hold. She bounced between the event's host, Darshak Sanghavi, director of the Centers for Medicare and Medicaid (CMS) Innovation Center's group on Preventive and Population Health Care Models, and each participant to ensure they saw their own potential role in 100M's mission. To facilitate the process, Stout's team had set up a dozen blank poster boards with titles like "Child Health," "Sustainable Financing," and "Mental Health," and participants migrated to areas of interest, switching every 10 minutes unless they were too engrossed to move on. I saw Estrus Tucker, an experienced facilitator from the Texas branch of the Center for Courage and Renewal, bringing together well-seasoned, uniformed officials with new program managers from agencies or government centers that I did not even know existed. For the day, hierarchies and legal counsel–approved positions were loosened in favor of meeting people who had become public servants for the common aim of building a healthier country. It was plain to see that the event was fulfilling a desire for a new set of organizational behaviors. In addition, the 100M Campaign team had tapped into a deep vein of latent energy in the form of motivated individuals from often massive organizations who shared information and analysis about the vastly different scales in which they work—local, regional, and national. If the opportunity or crisis were clear enough, the growing neighborhood-rooted, national network that the 100M Campaign represented could give a staid or embattled institution the ability to explore ways forward in the form of conversations it would otherwise never have.

Throughout the day, Derek Feeley, the CEO of the Institute for Healthcare Improvement, quietly observed from the back of the room. The IHI was founded in 1991 with a mission to help people and organizations mobilize around healthcare quality improvement. In 2008, they extended their well-known "triple aim" for healthcare to "population health," a term that has emerged in national discourse as a common touchstone for healthcare, public health, and community development. The ambiguity that results from overlapping usages of the same term by very different perspectives can lead to confusion and inaction, or it can spark extraordinary moments for entrepreneurship at individual, organizational, and collective action levels. The IHI and the 100M Healthier Lives Campaign it hosts are determined to cultivate the latter. From Feeley's perspective, the IHI "had to" proactively move its signature efforts in clinical healthcare improvement toward improving health writ large; hosting the 100M Campaign was its natural next step. For the VA, a federal agency under extraordinary pressure to act boldly from within the strictures of a thick bureaucracy, 100M represented a credible place to search for alternative ways to improve veteran health.

A COMMON AIM

By focusing upon a common aim—100 million measurably healthier lives by 2020, using a set of measures that would have to be adapted along the way and achieved through yet undefined sets of resources—participants would define a system of improving population health through the work of improving it together. The task of integrating healthcare and public health, or public health and community development, or community development and healthcare, poses unique challenges to each dyad. For example, healthcare systems and public health organizations approach the work of improving mental health in difficult-to-reach populations using compatible yet substantially different frameworks: available service delivery versus ensuring equitable access, respectively. Community development efforts to improve mental health may include building supportive housing and educating police forces; the former has deeper ties to healthcare delivery (by reducing readmissions), whereas the latter is a classic public health concern. The metrics of progress and paths of financing at the intersection of each dyad are substantively different. As national organizations turn to the work of integrating these pieces, the specific challenges of reconciling different perspectives lead to systemwide challenges that transcend any particular issue. This is where the 100M Campaign comes in.

Two specific problems that drew my attention, and ultimately led to my participation in 100M, are what David Erickson of the San Francisco Federal Reserve calls the "wrong pocket problem" and what his colleague Douglas Jutte calls the "wrong measures problem."[4]

The wrong pocket problem means that the significant social savings that accompany health improvement efforts in other sectors rarely accrue to the investor. For example, the Department of Transportation (DOT) may directly contribute to lower obesity rates in a neighborhood by improving mass transit, but the savings may accrue to the Department of Health and Human Services, which has no way to give DOT credit for its investment. This is not just a "high-level" issue. In a more local example, a community development finance institution or private developer may upgrade an affordable housing complex that emphasizes walkability, includes integrated job training, and even attract a healthy grocery store. However, a healthcare system that accrues the savings from reductions in hospitalizations in a low-income, elderly population (dually eligible for Medicare and Medicaid), probably does not even know about the housing or transportation investments that led to lower costs and better outcomes!

The consequence of the financial savings landing in the "wrong pocket" is that there is no feedback loop to strengthen the net benefit of an important partnership at the local level, which is reinforced by silos that extend all the way up to the structure of our federal departments. Bold private healthcare companies, like UnitedHealth Group, have used their considerable financial muscle to directly invest in affordable housing,[5] and former New York State health commissioner Nirav Shah did the same with state healthcare dollars.[6] However, without national integrators to reveal and communicate the structural fault lines these solutions address, it is often simply too hard to assemble the best alignments of interests at the neighborhood level.

The wrong measures problem is related. Traditional healthcare metrics focus on service delivery and actively limit the consideration of other paths to improving health. When a job-training program, for instance, is asked to contribute to neighborhood health improvement, they instinctually focus on employment opportunities that give people skills to participate in healthcare or public health organizations that focus on reducing obesity, diabetes, asthma, or infant mortality. They are understandably responding to a measurement environment that views clinical measures as proxies for health. However, they don't recognize that a high-quality job is a *direct* contributor to an individual's health improvement with strong benefits for the people around them. As a result, we lose the opportunity to measure and reinforce the importance of full, and fulfilling, employment—in all job sectors—in improving public health.

Ironically, the same problem stymies healthcare professionals who are trying to improve population health. We amplify the problem by reinforcing the belief that the primary drivers of a healthier life are clinical, without including, for instance, an individual's social connectivity as an important part of the equation. This oversight reduces the likelihood that ample healthcare resources will be proportionately applied. From both within and without healthcare systems, the wrong measures for living a healthier life are amplified in a feedback loop that biases toward traditional clinical data. This leads to more detailed measurement, which leads to better clinical data, which is then followed by more fine-grained measurement and qualitative analysis. Investment follows paths well trodden by data, rightly or wrongly. With the advent and excitement around big data analysis, the bias toward data-rich measures can inadvertently lead to the intense study and focus upon a limited or misguided set of measures, while dangerously neglecting others that are required for living a healthier life.

Although simple to state, problems of this nature are nearly impossible to solve in isolation and are heavily biased by the entity that is defining the problem. It is clear that a healthcare system is responsible for reducing errors within its hospitals, but who is responsible for reducing the number of people whose state of health that led to hospitalization could have been reliably prevented? After all, the data for the former is better, and the environment to measure and intervene upon it is more controlled. Furthermore, the initiative to reduce errors during hospitalization emerged, in part, from a patient safety movement that coincided with a healthcare quality improvement movement; consequently, hospitals have become the primary zone of problem solving when it comes to health improvement in general. However, to simultaneously reduce the number of patients who should not have been there in the first place, the nature of the solution depends upon the time scale being discussed, the perspectives involved, and the practical means of linking proposed actions together into a coherent plan. If multiple perspectives are given avenues for sharing the different ways they see the same situation, new opportunities for adaptive problem solving will inevitably emerge. Because such an exchange necessitates a national platform with the capacity to facilitate micro-interactions, this is precisely where nationally recognized organizations can come in to fill a new role beyond the execution of their mission, but within the embrace of their vision. IHI's mission—"Improve Health and Healthcare Worldwide"—comfortably accommodates its role in hosting 100M Healthier Lives. Rather than serve as leading front-runner of 100M Healthier Lives, they are ideally poised to be a backbone *integrator* of other national integrators, a coalition of coalitions. By adopting a process of cultural transformation from the beginning, the movement is fostering a rapidly growing community of change agents spanning the grassroots to the grasstops committed to unprecedented collaboration, an innovative and humble spirit of improvement, and systems transformation.

For this integration behavior to be systemic, there needs to be a mix of distinct but complementary organizations or coalitions that play a similar role, each driving together pieces of a much larger puzzle. Hundreds of organizations across the nation actively serve a variation on the purpose of integration; all issue- or constituency-oriented organizations that analyze, report on, and act upon policy, financing, data, and populations fit the bill. Here I will describe just five national integrators that paved the way for the formation of the 100M Healthier Lives Campaign, setting the stage for its work directly or indirectly: the National Academy of Medicine (formerly Institute of Medicine); the Dartmouth Institute for Health Policy and Clinical Practice; the American Public Health Association's Generation Public Health; Robert Wood Johnson Foundation's Commission to Build a Healthier America; and Douglas Jutte's Build Healthy Places Network.

NATIONAL INTEGRATORS

The Institute of Medicine

If ever there were an influential constituency about the state of affairs in medicine and healthcare, it would be the 2,000-plus members of the Institute of Medicine (IOM).[7] The *New York Times* has deemed it the "most esteemed and authoritative adviser on issues of health and medicine, and its reports can transform medical thinking around the world."[8] Members include academics, policy makers, private sector leaders in healthcare, as well as a substantial fraction (25 percent) who are required to be in professions other than health or healthcare. The elite and accomplished members actively participate in the development of expert-led, consensus-driven reports, which have regularly reflected large-scale course corrections in the theory and practice of biomedical research, clinical practice, healthcare delivery, and public health. They also focus on healthcare design-level issues, like efforts to bring "community health workers into the mainstream."[9]

The proliferation of measures for health, and the growing recognition of the wrong measures problem, led to the organization's release of *Vital Signs: Core Metrics for Health and Health Care Progress*: "To achieve better health at lower cost, all stakeholders—including health professionals, payers, policy makers, and members of the public—must be alert to the measures that matter most. What are the core measures that will yield the clearest understanding and focus on better health and well-being for Americans?"[10]

The suite of 15 "parsimonious measures" (see box 9.1) are a first approximation of ways to reduce measures *and* describe those that can be used by everyone. Although they clearly tilt toward classic measures of health and healthcare, they represent an authoritative shift to the neighborhood, where the real test of their durability will reside.

BOX 9.1
Vital Signs for Health and Healthcare

Vital Signs, a 2015 report from the Institute of Medicine, proposes a set of 15 core measures for health and health care.

1. Life Expectancy
2. Well-Being
3. Overweight and Obesity
4. Addictive Behavior
5. Unintended Pregnancy
6. Healthy Communities
7. Preventive Services
8. Care Access
9. Patient Safety
10. Evidence-Based Care
11. Care Match with Patient Goals
12. Personal Spending Burden
13. Population Spending Burden
14. Individual Engagement
15. Community Engagement

Vital Signs: Core Metrics for Health and Health Care Progress, Institute of Medicine Report, April 28, 2015, http://iom.nationalacademies.org/Reports/2015/Vital-Signs-Core-Metrics.aspx. See the interactive infographic available at http://resources.iom.edu/Infographics/VitalSigns/index.html?_ga=1.144556277.1144336317.1450821573.

Dartmouth Institute for Health Policy and Clinical Practice

Public health professionals have focused on the geography of health for over a century, particularly geographic disparities in health outcomes. The leaders at the Dartmouth Institute for Health Policy and Clinical Practice have applied similar frames to the clinical side of health, literally putting healthcare on the map. Through a series of landmark studies, Jonathan Wennberg, Elliott Fisher, and their colleagues have worked to understand and analyze the relationship between cost, healthcare utilization, and health outcomes. Their findings are complex and, at times, contested, but the productive collaboration of their current institute director, Elliott Fisher, with economists like Mark McClellan (Brookings), Jonathan Skinner (Dartmouth), and Amitabh Chandra (Harvard), have played a significant role in establishing the purpose and architecture of health reform, including delivery innovations like the accountable care organization (ACO). Now one of the most respected individual voices in healthcare, Fisher has begun to emphasize partnerships with community development and public health as the partner in improving population health: "The geographic communities in which people live and work have a profound effect on their health and the health care they receive. With strong support from national and local foundations, the Federal Reserve Bank, the Centers for Disease Control and Prevention, and others, a grassroots, community-level movement focused on establishing multisector, multistakeholder organizations to coordinate health-related initiatives has been increasing steadily for more than a decade."[11]

Through the process of inventing new methodologies for studying and measuring the links between healthcare and health in the neighborhood, it is also easier to identify where and how major disconnects—in both process and financing—need to be bridged. With the new partnership he describes above, Fisher and his contemporaries have envisioned moving beyond the ACO toward an accountable health community (AHC), a type of neighborhood-level integrator.[12] If this concept were adopted as widely as ACOs have been, the resulting AHCs would need regional support from all health sectors as well as pathways to accelerate their emergence on a national basis. In the process, both "wrong pocket" and "wrong measure" challenges would have to be directly addressed.

Generation Public Health

Whereas the Institute of Medicine requires at least 25 percent of its members to be in professions other than medicine or healthcare, the American Public Health Association (APHA) rapidly differentiated from the hospital-centric and professional associations of healthcare by diversifying its membership base early in its history. By maintaining a focus on the health of *all* people in *all* communities, it applies the broadest and most inclusive possible lens to health improvement, rooted in the geography of disparities and neighborhood-level contextual factors. Perhaps most notably, its tens of thousands of members worldwide are people like Donya Williams, public health practitioners who can drive local action and regional advocacy.

In 2014 the APHA developed a new flagship approach to bring its diverse membership together as a collective asset by issuing a challenge to members and partners to make America the healthiest nation in one generation. By focusing upon the full assembly of factors that lead to better health—climate and environment, food and nutrition, income, education, healthy behaviors and choices, neighborhoods, and healthcare—the public health community is able to build their own map of what leads to a healthier life, which they will do in partnership with the 100M Campaign.[13] Whereas the IOM's *Vital*

Signs are high-level conceptual measures and Fisher's accountable health communities are focused on the mechanics of neighborhood-level finances, outcomes, and governance, the Generation Public Health initiative is an umbrella for the public health community to create a national vision of what would need to be in place to achieve its ambitious big-data goals. The APHA's collective intelligence "big tent" approach purports to draw upon its members and partners to identify national gaps in action and missing information. Ideally, 100M will help the APHA tackle the challenge of building an integrated process that has enough focus to take advantage of its diversity.

Commission to Build a Healthier America

With 40 years' experience making philanthropic investments in health and healthcare, the Robert Wood Johnson Foundation (RWJF) launched the Commission to Build a Healthier America in 2008. Although RWJF's asset base sounds enormous—nearly $10 billion with about half a billion of spending per year—it has to carefully consider where to focus its energies to shape the arc and design of a $3 trillion health sector within its nonpartisan and national mandate. When the commission was launched in 2008, it focused upon a well-considered list of priorities, often reflecting high-impact investments or areas of diminished interest.[14] In the process of pursuing those goals, its grantees demonstrated how more-integrated approaches, like the grassroots organizing work of ISAIAH that purposefully linked transportation and health, are crucial to its mission. By 2014, RWJF had honed its message to focus on early childhood development, which requires the integration of community development, public health, and healthcare in a more textured way. More than a list of things to do, it was an appeal to core American values, making things right for another generation, and building a culture of health that *definitively* includes thinking from many perspectives at once.

Their observations were striking and influential (see box 9.2), amplifying what we know and stressing that we must immediately take action, and do so in a way that addresses the growing inequality of opportunity: "Unless we act now, our nation will continue to fall farther behind, putting our health, economic prosperity, and national security at even greater risk. ... Low-income children must have the same opportunities to be healthy as all children in America, no matter where they live. Leaving them behind would put our nation's well-being and prosperity at great peril."[15] Across the country and political spectrum, pre-kindergarten education has become a national rallying cry, oftentimes directly limited by the impact of insidious growth in healthcare spending on local budgets. By bringing attention to our nation's children, the future of our global competitiveness as a nation, the commission struck a national chord with deep neighborhood roots.

As a result, RWJF has invested in the 100M Healthier Lives Campaign through an initiative called Spreading Community Accelerators through Learning and Evaluation (SCALE). The hope is that it will be a means to accelerate the growth and connectivity of many overlapping and complementary national networks—to bend a long arc of healthcare reform ahead of us toward a more comprehensive definition of health.

BOX 9.2
The Toll of Poor Health

On our children: 1 in 3 children is overweight or obese.

On our young adults: 3 in 4 Americans ages 17 to 24 are ineligible to serve in the U.S. military, primarily because they are inadequately educated, have criminal records, or are physically unfit.

On our economy: Poor health results in the U.S. economy losing $576 billion a year, with 39 percent, or $227 billion, of those losses due to lost productivity from employees who are ill.

On our national investments: Medicare would save billions of dollars if every state performed as well as the top-performing states in key measures of health.

On poverty and racism: More than one-fifth of all U.S. children live in poor families, and nearly half of black children live in particularly unhealthy areas of concentrated poverty.

On our neighborhoods: 1 out of 5 Americans live in unhealthy neighborhoods with limited employment, low-quality housing, pollution, few opportunities for a healthy diet and physical activity.

Modified from "Beyond Health Care: New Directions to a Healthier America," Robert Wood Johnson Foundation, April 2009, http://www.rwjf.org/content/dam/farm/reports /reports/2009/rwjf40483.

Build Healthy Places Network

In 2014, RWJF announced its strategic shift to "building a culture of health," which includes cultivating a shared vision for what this means, building demand for this shared vision across America, and discovering and investing in the solutions that emerge.[16] With a particular emphasis on boundary-spanning partnerships, RWJF invested in the Build Healthy Places Network, which works at the intersection of community development, public health, and healthcare to accomplish three goals: (1) highlight examples of success that feature complex investments of more than one type, particularly where the role of a local integrator clearly emerges; (2) concentrate on bridging the gap between community development and the healthcare sector, with a particular emphasis on childhood development as a means to focus local attention; and (3) build a measurement portal that helps people across neighborhoods assign the right metrics to financial and health impacts. Douglas Jutte, a pediatrician and public health practitioner who described the "wrong measures" problem to me, leads the network. As a scholar, he has compared the health impacts on children who live in deteriorating public housing versus those who live in redeveloped housing. He found that children who live in the former are 39 percent more likely to have repeat healthcare visits over the course of a year.[17]

This level of evidence is frustratingly below the threshold needed to redirect the spending of healthcare dollars. Even if such spending adjustments were possible, most places across the nation would not know how to develop effective and efficient relationships between real estate development, healthcare, and public health; nor would they know how to rigorously measure its impact so that confidence in this link could be reinforced. To prepare neighborhoods to see the opportunities for integrating multiple sectors, and know what to do when they emerge, Jutte's network is scouring the country for places that are actively addressing the wrong pocket problem, and sharing their methods, mindset, and approach.

For example, Maggie Super Church of the Healthy Neighborhoods Equity Fund in Boston recognized that targeted investments in distressed blocks, where people are more likely to be in poor health, could drive financial returns in a manner that can be shared beyond the immediate beneficiaries in terms of improved health, public revenue base, environmental impact, and economic mobility.[18] She analyzes potential investments against a set of parsimonious and evidence-based public health quality requirements that her organization has developed and places particular emphasis on functional requirements (e.g., that new development should improve walkability). By helping investors recognize the connection between community development and local public health, Church strives to raise awareness of their integral role in building the local public health system's architecture.

Jutte's home base in California has had the consistent support of the California Endowment's Healthy Communities fund, which has created a portfolio of "bright spots" that serve as idea sources for others in the growing network. Jutte's vision is national in scope, but like all other national initiatives, has a stronger presence in some places than others.

A Network of National and Local Integrators

At some point, individuals who lead regional and national networks come into contact with each other: through common funders, shared challenges, or the same constituents. This is what makes the world of health improvement actors feel small for some well-recognized individuals, like Mark McClellan or Rebecca Onie (both RWJF commissioners), vast but comprehensible to most practitioners who work in a particular subarea of health, and impossibly distant for a person in his or her own neighborhood. In this sense, Stout's 100M Healthier Lives Campaign has one overarching goal, which is to create a small world out of vast, disconnected networks and ensure that wherever you are in the country, as a person, patient, practitioner, or organization leader, you can plug in and search them for support and guidance, while contributing your own. Under the right conditions, this even has an appeal for large institutions like the VHA that seem like they are already everywhere but suffer from dangerously low-quality connections.

For the VHA, 100M offers the chance to channel the VHA's assets and relationships beyond hospital or clinic-centric services so it can help veterans assemble the diverse pathways to healthier lives available to them in their neighborhoods. Using the tools 100M offers, the government agency can observe what works and then efficiently amplify support in those areas while commissioning support where it is lacking, all without accidentally suppressing smaller, independent efforts that are working just fine at the neighborhood level.

INTEGRATION FOR THE COMMON GOOD

No transformation of American healthcare can be complete without the participation of the federal government. Situated in the bunkerlike Hubert H. Humphrey Building on Capitol Hill, the Department of Health and Human Services (HHS) has been the target of nearly continuous political ire from across the political spectrum for its central role in conceiving, implementing, and then defending the ACA. Since even before the Medicaid and Medicare amendments were added to the Social Security Act in 1965, the role of this federal agency (and its predecessors) has been the subject of scrutiny, refinement, and nearly continuous redesign. In fiscal year 2015, its budget was just a hair over $1 trillion,[19] with 90 percent residing in the Centers for Medicare and Medicaid Services (nearly double 2005's numbers). Just for comparison to its other well-known subdivisions, 3 percent of the total budget goes to the National Institutes of Health, 0.6 percent goes to the Centers for Disease Control, and 0.2 percent goes to the Food and Drug Administration. The department's overwhelming responsibility is to healthcare, which is both an investment in the health of our nation and a ballooning fiscal obligation. We know, for instance, that Medicaid for children reduces the need for hospitalizations and emergency department visits later in life, particularly in kids who live in low-income neighborhoods.[20] We also know that the number of elderly who live beyond the age of 65 in our country has gone from 20 percent at the beginning of the 20th century to greater than 80 percent today,[21] with support for Medicare strong among seniors.[22]

Americans have consistently supported the expansion of healthcare coverage for decades, felt buyer's remorse shortly after doing so, and regained their enthusiasm in time for the next expansionist push. As a result, HHS's focus has been nearly completely dominated by the management of its considerable role in both directly setting the terms of public healthcare financing and influencing private sector trends. Even today, as the growth in healthcare delivery–related expenditures slows, the prices of new pharmaceutical products are rising at an alarming rate, foreshadowing a new battle to give HHS the ability to negotiate for bulk purchase of drugs on behalf of taxpayers. This is all to say that HHS's role in America's economic and fiscal policy will continue to grow, competing with its stated role in health improvement. Under this strain and focus, the public health and neighborhood health improvement functions at the federal, state, and local levels will have even less officially sanctioned room to invest in innovative approaches to health improvement, hampered by the economic dominance of healthcare systems they see as a threat rather than as a resource to draw upon.

In the face of these mounting constraints and tensions, the growing mesh of national integrator organizations, like those described above, is arguably our best bet for keeping our collective focus trained on how Americans will live healthier lives. The actions of many motivated individuals within government, including HHS, are helping these institutions make great strides in this direction. Three government employees in particular, Peggy Honoré of HHS, Darshak Sanghavi of CMMI, and David Erickson of the Federal Reserve, whom I met through the 100M Healthier Lives Campaign, showed me how the federal government can be an effective national integrator. All three of them have minimal if any budgetary power within titanic bureaucracies, which leads them to think creatively, informally, and with an eye for the abundance of talent and resources outside, rather than the relative scarcity within.

Peggy Honoré

Within HHS, Peggy Honoré is director of the Public Health System, Finance, and Quality Program in the office of the assistant secretary of health. Honoré sees her department's role as one of "building self-awareness." Advocating for a systematic view of public health, in which local aims are well defined, achieved, and measured, she believes the federal government's role should be one of enabler and accelerator rather than an entity that passes down uniform regulations and supplies from on high.

"I had a conversation with someone in the Mississippi delta region, and her comment to me was, 'I wish the federal government would send some people down here to fix our teenage pregnancy problem.' I said, 'Can you tell me that again? What can the government deploy for that?!' That's a problem with local context, and it needs local people to think it through, before we leap in with some right answer we don't have."[23]

Far from thinking that HHS has no role in teenage pregnancy, Honoré is relentlessly focused on how to build local awareness that America's places— whether they are neighborhoods, counties, or rural communities—are the new "marquee platforms" of the public health systems she envisions to address these sorts of complex issues. This is why forming a strong collaboration with the 100 Million Healthier Lives Campaign was so attractive for her. She understood that for most complicated challenges to health, there can be no single leader: the public health system she envisions is a boundary-spanning, collaborative system, where embedding a strong tradition of distributed, rather than central, decision-making is the key to improvement. Honoré is widely considered to be a strong champion of a public health *system*, which aims to unify the immense breadth of activity that influences health across multiple sectors. When she uses the term "public health system," it is clear that she is not simply speaking about *what* ought to be done, but *how* a system emerges from the incredible array of activities that can be considered part of improving the health of Americans.

In 2010, HHS produced its Healthy People 2020 agenda, which was launched to monitor progress in four areas: general health status, health-related quality of life and well-being, determinants of health, and disparities of health. With most of HHS preoccupied with the economic realities of managing a staggering healthcare budgetary outlay, the Healthy People 2020 agenda seems secondary at best. But in the realms of public health and community activism, an HHS agenda of this kind is momentous. For her persistent and practical efforts to build a systems view of public health, the APHA recognized Honoré's contributions to public health administration in 2013. When the 100M Healthier Lives Campaign came up, she immediately saw that its extensive network provided an opportunity to promulgate a vision of public health as the premier collaborator within a neighborhood, enriched with expertise in finance, quality, and safety.

Darshak Sanghavi

Even though Honoré works within the same federal department—the same building even—as Darshak Sanghavi, they actually only met through a 100M Campaign event in 2014. Sanghavi had joined CMMI that year to advance its stalled efforts to build an effective and financially viable approach to shifting healthcare dollars to preventive and population health. Like Douglas Jutte and Don Berwick, both pediatricians by training, Sanghavi viewed healthcare through the eyes of the children who came to see him as patients. Through the lens of a child's needs, Sanghavi naturally sought solutions beyond healthcare, and beyond its specializing forces. Even though he was training as a pediatric cardiologist, a specialist, he knew that even if his patients received fantastic care, they would need integrated and self-reinforcing support systems to help them develop to their full potential. Most pediatricians know that well before a child turns 18 and becomes an independent adult with legal decision-making capacity, their trajectory of development as a person is loosely[24] predictable across many integrated dimensions: health, education, economic opportunity, social mobility, etc. No child's path is fixed at birth, but the basic building blocks of mental and physical development are either rapidly improving or falling dangerously behind. They know that in a child's development, barricades between healthcare, public health, and community development are actively dangerous.

Prior to joining the federal government, Sanghavi was the Merkin Fellow for Finance Reform and Clinical Leadership and Managing Director for Economic Studies at the Center for Health Policy, while still practicing as a cardiac pediatrician. When Sanghavi initially joined CMMI, he was thinking about ways to solve the wrong pocket/wrong measure problem, which in his field can be exemplified by a situation in which the solution to a child's worsening asthma condition may not be more medication but rather removal of mold from his or her home. After months spent figuring out the federal government while having hundreds of conversations about how to move forward, he began to work with his team to make the accountable health communities (AHCs) concept a reality. They were building upon the groundwork that Elliott Fisher's group at the Dartmouth Institute had laid for accountable care organizations (ACOs) and early descriptions of its extensions in the community.[25]

In theory, CMMI's mandate is simple: if they can show that an alternative payment model saves money and improves health, it can become a federally allowable use of healthcare dollars without further congressional approval. In reality, health improvement is extremely difficult to prove given the stringent evidentiary and financial requirements of HHS's budget office. To date, only one CMMI program, the ACO, has passed muster, despite several setbacks. In hopes of replicating the ACO model's successful passage through CMMI hurdles, Sanghavi reached into the 100M Healthier Lives Campaign networks for initial reactions, feedback, and concept development. Next, he hosted the 100 Million Healthier Lives Summit in Baltimore later that year—the same gathering where VHA director Regan Crump called upon interested participants to help his department's 20 million veterans. Like all participants in 100M, Sanghavi recognizes that sometimes the best ideas are not waiting to be invented so much as waiting to be effectively spread and scaled across the nation. The AHC concept echoes the community "hub" idea, the brainchild of community health worker advocate Mark Redding, whose presence at the summit reinforced the collaborative nature of the 100M Campaign. The 100M Campaign team drew participants' attention to Jutte's Build Healthy Places Network, which could prove instrumental in spreading the ACO concept. And although Erickson could not attend, his persistent national message that the Federal Reserve system was a bridge to the approximately $200 billion community development industry was readily heard.[26]

David Erickson

The Federal Reserve system's community development mandate sits on the far periphery of its headline role in defining our nation's monetary policy—maximizing employment, stabilizing prices (colloquially referred to as managing inflation), and moderating long-term interest rates as necessary.[27] As described in part 1, community development corporations (CDCs) and financing institutions (CDFIs) arose after the passage of the 1973 Community Reinvestment Act (CRA), with an initial focus on improving access to credit markets and banking services in underserved areas and shifting the affordable housing production responsibility from the Department of Housing and Urban Development to a mesh of local intermediaries.

Even though this function is most closely associated with the Federal Reserve's community development role, Erickson points out that its mission is not limited to real estate and banking, but instead encompasses the entire process of community development. This necessarily includes the health of the people involved. The Primary Care Development Corporation (PCDC), founded in 1993 and headquartered in New York City, has bridged the traditional world of CDCs and healthcare by leveraging $515 million to improve access to care for 765,000 patients, training an estimated 7,000 healthcare workers in more than one million square feet of upgraded space for neighborhood-based primary care clinics.[28] Instead of taking a dollar and putting it directly into healthcare services, PCDC makes directed loans and capital investments to build the infrastructure for primary care, including community health centers in underserved areas. PCDC is a step in the right direction. However, Erickson believes that by truly integrating the financial and operational experience of the healthcare sector and community development industry, the nation could take a leap forward.

Erickson is the director of the Center for Community Development Investments at the Federal Reserve Bank of San Francisco. He has played an instrumental national role in bringing the world of community development and health improvement together. He edits the Federal Reserve journal *Community Development Investment Review* and has written an authoritative history of community development in *The Housing Policy Revolution: Networks and Neighborhoods*. Most importantly, he is a relentless organizer, evangelist, and problem solver, bridging the worlds of social impact investing, economic policy, and community development with health. In 2014, I reached out to him in my new capacity as organizer of the "network hub" on sustainable business models and financing for the 100M Healthier Lives Campaign. His challenge as an integrator is a tough one. He must actively help his constituency—housing development, mostly—shift beyond thinking about community development only in terms of physical infrastructure, and at the same time orient them to the rapidly evolving world of population health improvement. Through work with RWJF, he has homed in on a gateway area of collaboration between CDFIs and primary care: childhood health and development.

It is rare to find one person who commands such a breadth of relationships and expertise; Erickson's source of deep insight into how the world of the Fed bears upon the health of America's children comes from another relationship: Jutte, his partner, who in turn brings Erickson's expertise and networks to bear upon the Build Healthy Places Network.

Collectively, these individuals represent the type of creativity, drive, and diversity of knowledge needed to move the behemoth of federal healthcare forward.

A CAMPAIGN TO BUILD A NETWORK OF RELATIONSHIPS

Sometimes the ability to drive historically disconnected and substantively differentiated areas of work emerges from the fortuitous relationship between a pair of people who can speak for the vision of their respective worlds. It is not uncommon in politics or media to see talented couples or long-term friends who forged their personal relationships long before professional interests arose as powerful drivers of creativity and progress. This type of synergy is well represented by Erickson and Jutte. In a conversation I had with the couple about where the 100M Campaign fit into the landscape they saw, I heard them artfully represent the complexities of integrating two dense national networks. Where Jutte is more optimistic about progress toward integrating the aims of the healthcare and community development sectors, Erickson expresses a hint of pessimism. Jutte points out that of the 8–10 major national CDFIs, all have incorporated health into their missions. Because of this, he's hopeful about a solution to the "wrong pocket" problem that Erickson articulates. Erickson, who knows these networks better, sees that his colleagues remain rooted in their skills as investors of capital, usually with a building like a clinic or hospital in mind; their "health lens" typically involves clinicians inside of this building providing classic healthcare service. This mindset only reinforces the "wrong measures" problem that the 100M Campaign is meant to help resolve.

In *Investing in What Works for America's Communities*, Erickson and his co-authors explore dozens of examples of solving the "wrong pocket" problem. In a companion volume called *What Counts: Harnessing Data for America's Communities*, the authors describe cogent solutions to the "wrong measures" problem.[29] Although there are general strategies and tools, the work of actually addressing these issues is necessarily specific to each of our country's neighborhoods. With approximately 200,000 neighborhoods,[30] there are undoubtedly repeating motifs of challenges and solutions, but the work of discovering and leading the process of addressing them remains unique to each. To even *begin* to understand if there are any general principles that could be advanced in common across regions, states, or even the nation, we need an integrated network of neighborhood-level problem solvers who can share their insights and issues with their peers across the country: an Internet of neighborhoods, to integrate bits of insights as they emerge, while enabling solutions that work to rapidly spread and scale across the nation.

For the 100M Campaign to achieve its goal, it has to allow traditionally disconnected silos to see themselves as part of an integrated future: an "unprecedented collaboration of change agents who are pursuing an unprecedented result."[31] Stout elaborates further by saying that an unprecedented collaboration includes the "joy, relationships and structures to create and sustain it + innovative, at scale improvement + systems transformation." These are driven by core goals: (1) create a healthcare system that's good at health and good at care; (2) build bridges between healthcare, community, public health, and social service systems; (3) create healthy communities; (4) create peer to-peer support systems; (5) create enabling conditions; and (6) develop new mindsets. Its boldest claim is that somewhere in the country, the substance of each of these strategies is already among us, or has the potential to rapidly emerge with support.

For 100M, its challenge is a variant on an adage commonly attributed to William Gibson: "the future is already here—it is just not evenly distributed."

10

SCALE at the Speed of Relationships

The type of coordination required to change a whole neighborhood . . .
requires bringing together dozens of institutions and thousands
of people inside and outside a community . . . It is a millipede with
hundreds of legs.
—Investing in What Works for America's Communities

SCALE: LEARNING HOW NEIGHBORHOODS LEARN

After the October 2014 Escape Velocity event, hundreds of new groups joined the 100M Campaign. It seemed that if a group joined from Wisconsin, then a clump of other organizations in the region would follow. If a group joined with expertise in the patient experience, then a clump of their peer organizations would follow. If a large insurer joined the discussion, then employees or personally interested people from other companies would inquire about the campaign. Multiple philanthropic foundations took note and saw opportunities to bring the health-related initiatives they had been supporting into a bigger arena. This avalanche of interest was triggered by a simple request: do you have something to offer toward the "audacious goal" of 100 million healthier lives?

Without any promise of funding or money, people across the country resoundingly affirmed the notion that they had a piece of a larger puzzle and were looking for ways to build upon what they had. Despite the radically different sizes and types of organizations that were participating in the 100M Campaign—from Ascension Healthcare to the United States Air Force to the Alaska Native Medical Center—their common focus was on how places across the country—from regions to bases to neighborhoods and towns— could take a leap forward in health improvement. All along the way, group members who had expertise in measuring progress, resource planning, and tracking impact were put in productive tension with those who had ample experience in activating social movements that had an energy of their own.

The core team had to begin thinking about how this energy would be practically channeled to support real places. They devised SCALE—Spreading Community Accelerators through Learning and Evaluation—with the backing of the Robert Wood Johnson Foundation, to create a learning network of places across the country that wanted to accelerate and improve upon their early efforts to better the health of their neighbors. Since levels of experience in defining common aims, paths to improvement, and sustainable financing varied considerably, the network included a few experienced "mentors" and a community of motivated "pacesetters" who wanted to grow to be effective mentors. While the 100M team cultivated hubs of topical support (e.g., "how do you improve the health of children?"; "how should housing be designed to support the elderly?") and regional connectivity (e.g., aligned state and regional initiatives), the SCALE initiative aimed to test how a national backbone of experienced organizations could directly provide support for improvement in pacesetters in a way that could be financially sustained and scaled as the network grew. The 100M Campaign focused upon increasing the number and density of diverse connections, and SCALE would improve their quality and relevance to street-level activities. Put another way, as the 100M Campaign developed an overarching *structure*, SCALE would develop its *logic*: the core principles that would guide decision-making for the campaign. Together they would yield a national neighborhood-level health improvement network.

The upcoming gathering of the 100M Campaign members in Grapevine, Texas, scheduled for March 2015, would provide an opportunity to get SCALE off the ground. This meant there was only about two months, starting from the beginning of 2015, to get the word out. They invited members of the campaign's guiding coalition to select the pacesetters and mentors. The core team worried that the campaign would not be able to get the word out in time, and if they did, there would not be enough places across the country that would be ready to participate. They were wrong, and by the time the group was assembled in Grapevine, they had 175 high-potential applications from across the country. In one of the many side conference rooms, I joined the intense team that would select the 20 pacesetters and a smaller number of mentors that would seed the network.

The places that applied to be part of SCALE are a cross section of America: rural, urban, and every shade in between; metropolitan regions to tiny towns; predominantly one-community places to areas with many communities that had spent years devising ways to share power. Many were already members of regional or national improvement networks, and networks of networks, like Community Solutions, Communities Joined in Action, and the Collaborative Health Network; but a remarkable number were not. The financial incentives to apply were miniscule: pacesetters were given enough money to hire one person and to bring a team of leaders and community members with lived experience to participate in the Community Health Improvement Academy that was being developed as a learning platform for SCALE and the broader 100M Campaign. Mentors were simply given the opportunity to share their experience. Even with minimal outreach, the demand to be connected was considerable.

The chief purpose of the Community Health Improvement Academy is to support representatives from the SCALE pacesetters themselves. Once the right measures and accountability terms are determined, how can the pacesetter representative incorporate these into her skills and scaffolds of support back home in the neighborhood?

Two terms, "skills" and "scaffolds" are worth explaining in more detail. In a large body of work by James Heckman and his colleagues, expounded upon in a paper entitled "The Economics of Human Development and Social Mobility," they state that skills "are multiple in nature and encompass cognition, personality, preference parameters, as well as health. Skills are capacities to act . . . they shape expectations, constraints, and information. More capacities enlarge agent choice sets."[1] To put this in plain language, building multiple skills and identifying gaps in skills is crucial to enabling a person to see opportunities and navigate challenges in day-to-day life. A complementary concept is a "scaffold," or "an adaptive interactive strategy that recognizes the current capacities of the trainee and guides him/her to further learning." In short, skills should be built within scaffolds that guide those skills forward. These concepts can be useful to a group of neighborhood organizations that have never worked together toward a common aim when they get ready to take their first steps.

To translate this back to SCALE, mentors were chosen because they had used a variety of collaborative scaffolds and identified skills they needed to achieve their goals. They also had an explicit interest in teaching what they had learned with pacesetters because they believed that they would also learn more through a self-reflective process. All the while, the SCALE pacesetter communities have been setting direction on the aims that matter to them, while being exposed to a broader set of possible determinants that may lead to improvement in the aims themselves (e.g., taking equity into consideration, or adjusting a short-term goal so a medium-term one is possible). Since the precise set of skills and scaffolds required are not known, success depends upon how effectively the entire SCALE network can collaborate to find innovative solutions and come to rough consensus on the most effective ones that the academy should promulgate.

At the Community Health Improvement Academy, representatives from participating organizations learn an approach from the MIT Center for Collective Intelligence called a Collaborative Innovation Network (COIN),[2] a process that has been used by a national consortium of child health organizations to address the alarmingly high infant mortality rates in many parts of the country.[3] Peter Gloor, an MIT scientist who described COIN based upon his research on effective virtual collaborative structures, helps contextualize why this approach would be useful for the 100M Campaign: "COIN are self-organizing groups of highly motivated individuals working together towards a common goal not because of orders from their superiors, but because the members of a COIN share the same goal and are convinced of their common cause."[4]

These principles of self-organization and motivation toward a common goal describe the essence of the entire 100M Campaign effort, not just the pacesetters who are members of SCALE. As a result, this basic structure is echoed across many levels of the campaign, ranging from how topical hubs operate to how a regional hub, like New York City, functions. Without being dogmatic, these models enable representatives from the pacesetters to begin to recognize this form of teamwork around them and lead a successful collaborative process. What results is a "super organization" that transcends organizational boundaries because it is easy to join a COIN that reflects and advances a shared interest (e.g., a child health organization would join a COIN on a relevant topic, and a mentor organization would join a regional COIN to interact with fellow mentors and pacesetters alike). By disseminating a core set of common concepts at SCALE academy, its nascent network of pacesetters can begin to discern effective processes and build upon them, setting the stage for further spread.

The purpose of SCALE as a formative learning opportunity for the entire campaign was clear. Abe Wandersman, who leads the evaluation of the initiative, sees it as a bridge to the momentum that was growing in the broader 100M Campaign, rather than an isolated experiment or pilot project: "Learning what it takes to ignite and sustain peer-to-peer support and learning among and between communities will yield new strategies that all communities can tap into. The hope is that determining best practices by communities will add to data-informed decision-making about health, and will have a snowball effect on the journey toward widespread improvement."[5]

IMPROVING FROM THE INSIDE OUT

SCALE is built on a number of basic principles that govern interactions between members of the network. These principles facilitate the horizontal exchange of ideas across groups. For example, rather than relying on an executive committee or leadership to decide on a small group of "best" ideas to disseminate downward, groups are at liberty to choose for themselves what new ideas they wish to incorporate from each other.

The first principle is a fundamental agreement on the importance of embracing individuals in the neighborhood as essential to the process of building healthier communities. On conference calls that served as the main medium to organize the 100M Campaign across the country, it was not uncommon to hear people evoke the name of Elinor Ostrom to convey their own understanding of what the campaign would accomplish at the neighborhood level. Ostrom's work extended the concept of "polycentric governance" to explain how people maintained trust and accountability where common pooled resources (CPR)—water, forests, municipal resources—were at stake. This included the utilization of "cheap talk," as discussed in chapter 3. On the day she died in June 2012, her last piece, "Green from the Grassroots," was published. In it, she said, "Setting goals can overcome inertia, but everyone must have a stake in establishing them: countries, states, cities, organizations, companies, and people everywhere. Success will hinge on developing many overlapping policies to achieve the goals."[6] By evoking Ostrom, the campaign privileges the notion that the people within neighborhoods have significant insight into and intrinsic motivation for improving their own health, just as a City Health Works health coach would elicit using MI.

As Ostrom noted in her 2009 Nobel Prize speech, she believes in change initiated from the inside out:

> When analysts perceive the human beings they model as being trapped inside perverse situations, they then assume that other human beings external to those involved—scholars and public officials—are able to analyze the situation, ascertain why counterproductive outcomes are reached, and posit what changes in the rules-in-use will enable participants to improve outcomes. Then, external officials are expected to impose an optimal set of rules on those individuals involved. It is assumed that the momentum for change must come from outside the situation rather than from the self-reflection and creativity of those within a situation to restructure their own patterns of interaction.[7]

This is the same assumption that led the public health experts encountered in part 1 to operate without active co-development with the neighborhood's many communities.

Her work on polycentric governance started with the premise that people do not always act as classically self-interested beings, particularly where common-pool resources like forests or water are concerned. Instead they devise ways to balance many interests and perspectives (hence, polycentric) using implicit rules that she endeavored to make explicit. The work she did to understand the design of these governance systems can be considered the conceptual predecessor of Mark Kramer and John Kania's *collective impact* model, which involves "a centralized infrastructure, a dedicated staff, and a structured process that leads to a common agenda, shared measurement, continuous communication, and mutually reinforcing activities among all participants." This model forms the core of SCALE's logic. The basic premise is that "large-scale social change comes from better cross-sector coordination rather than from the isolated intervention of individual organizations."[8]

Ostrom provides descriptions of the structures used to create mutual accountability in situations that require polycentric governance (see box 10.1). But she leaves open the question of how these structures are arrived at in the first place: how do you take a group that wants to work collaboratively and help it to create true polycentric structures? This question is addressed by the theory of *collective impact*. The work of collective impact focuses on

---

BOX 10.1
Design Principles for Polycentric Governance

1A. *User Boundaries*: Clear and locally understood boundaries between legitimate users and nonusers are present.

1B. *Resource Boundaries*: Clear boundaries that separate a specific common-pool resource from a larger social-ecological system are present.

2A. *Congruence with Local Conditions*: Appropriation and provision rules are congruent with local social and environmental conditions.

2B. *Appropriation and Provision*: Appropriation rules are congruent with provision rules; the distribution of costs is proportional to the distribution of benefits.

3. *Collective Choice Arrangements*: Most individuals affected by a resource regime are authorized to participate in making and modifying its rules.

4A. *Monitoring Users*: Individuals who are accountable to or are the users monitor the appropriation and provision levels of the users.

4B. *Monitoring the Resource*: Individuals who are accountable to or are the users monitor the condition of the resource.

5. *Graduated Sanctions*: Sanctions for rule violations start very low but become stronger if a user repeatedly violates a rule.

6. *Conflict Resolution Mechanisms*: Rapid, low-cost, local arenas exist for resolving conflicts among users or with officials.

7. *Minimal Recognition of Rights*: The rights of local users to make their own rules are recognized by the government.

8. *Nested Enterprises*: When a common-pool resource is closely connected to a larger social-ecological system, governance activities are organized in multiple nested layers.

Elinor Ostrom, "Beyond Markets and States: Polycentric Governance of Complex Economic Systems," *American Economic Review* 100 (2010): 1–33, http://bnp.binghamton.edu/wp-content/uploads/2011/06/Ostrom-2010-Polycentric-Governance.pdf.

---

the need for a group to take on certain properties that have to do with how it functions, not what its goals are. In technical language, these properties are known as the *logic* of a system: they describe how a system needs to be—whether it must be of a certain quality, or flexibility, or reliability—in order to move toward its goals. This is the work of 100M: to define how groups collaborate toward a continuously refined goal of health.

The 100M Campaign isn't the only one to adopt a collective impact framework. These ideas form the basis of the accountable health communities (AHCs), which Fisher and his colleagues from the Dartmouth Institute for Health Policy and Clinical Practice describe as having the following ingredients: "(1) a coordinating (i.e., backbone) organization that mobilizes diverse cross-sector leadership to (2) set a common agenda and (3) pursue mutually reinforcing activities supported by (4) continuous communication to build trust and relationships and (5) shared measurement systems."[9]

When I think of my own neighborhood in Harlem, the thought of co-designing this neighborhood-level health system with the hundreds of organizations and thousands of people who live within it is daunting. Each of the pacesetters in SCALE were chosen for having had some experience in working through the conversations needed for successful co-design, whereas mentors had demonstrated a level of conscious expertise in achieving collaborative outcomes that they could share with others. SCALE is designed to bring these insights into productive focus, to help the pacesetters create a neighborhood-level health improvement system that could improve from the inside out. Imagine an alternative where every neighborhood suddenly had all of the organizations mentioned in part 2 imposed on them as externally sponsored interventions. Despite the individual promise of the groups, there would inevitably be questions about how they relate to each other and existing organizations, set boundaries of mutual responsibility, resolve conflicts as tensions surfaced, and so on. Most neighborhoods do not have all the ingredients to support productive conversations about how all of their assets interact while balancing self-interest and collective benefit. They may not even know how to initiate such a conversation in the first place, despite having clear aspirations if they did.

SCALE NET

Each of the 175 places that applied to be part of SCALE had a unique theory of change—a set of assumptions they held about how their neighbors would be able to lead healthier lives. They defined "healthier lives" in specific ways, and their assumptions reflected their sense of how to get there based upon what they had, and the support and guidance they felt they needed.

In the traditional model, a public health organization would define a set of health priorities for a region based upon epidemiological data, devise interventions, and construct a set of measures to track the impact of these interventions. In this conventional scenario each neighborhood's theory of change would vanish as a common set of measures was imposed across many places. So too would the neighborhood's ability to test their assumptions, change their strategy based upon data-informed feedback, and learn the evidence in the process. Their intrinsic motivation to act would likely suffer, and the status quo of externally defined aims would persist.

Instead of setting priorities at the top and vertically disseminating tools to achieve them, SCALE and 100M are based on the idea that priorities can be set locally, and ideas to fulfill those goals can be spread *horizontally*. This is achieved through exchange: of ideas, insights, and information. Within the network of organizations that constitute 100M, exchange is facilitated by a universally adopted set of guidelines for the creation, strengthening, and maintenance of relationships based on mutual opportunity and motivation.

But in order for redesign of the healthcare system to be truly successful, these principles of exchange must be adopted in all aspects of the system. Today, information about health or healthcare measures goes into electronic health records or public health databases, and rarely makes its way back out. In EHRs, the data is carefully protected and difficult for individuals to retrieve. The system makes it nearly impossible for an individual to easily contribute to advance neighborhood-level initiatives. Similarly, in public health databases, it is impossible to work backward from aggregated statistics to discover the assemblies of social networks and organizations that yielded the result. Perhaps as a result, US government agencies and foundations have commissioned reports to guide the future of our health data architecture.[10] For healthcare system–based EHRs, which are at the center of the federal discussion, there are growing efforts to do simple things with the individual healthcare data locked within, such as allow it to be transportable to and interoperable with any other healthcare system. One important effort called Open Notes enables patients to be active discussants in their own care.[11] The fact that this project *is* cutting edge indicates how distant our healthcare data architecture is from being usable by individuals, much less for neighborhood-level health improvement efforts.

As we reconsider how information is exchanged, we must take into account not only *how* data is shared, but *what* data is considered worth collecting and sharing. "Big data" definitely has its place: it allows analytics to discern insights or patterns from large amounts of information, much like what PCCI (Parkland Center for Clinical Innovation) does to anticipate at-risk populations; the score a person receives reflects systemic risk, not their individual trajectory. However, if an individual like Ray wanted feedback on how to live a healthier life as it happened, or exchange insights that worked with his neighbors, big data in this format would be useless without substantial skill and resource. Similarly, if Harlem organized as an accountable health community and defined its own goals and pathways for action, it would find that a rigidly structured big data framework would not help if it wanted to exchange insights about processes that worked with neighborhoods across the country who were undertaking a similar (but not exactly the same) path to improvement.

Instead, we need more "small data": granular-level insights that improve the heuristics—the practical problem-solving approaches—of individuals, organizations, and entire neighborhoods. This context-sensitive feedback isn't just about measurements or statistics, it is about a mindset of improvement that builds from where any one person or place is currently. The difference between "big data" and "small data" is not the amount of information, but rather the *type* of insight they aim to provide. For SCALE, a small-data mindset would be the key to identifying person-centric innovations in living a healthier life within a neighborhood, which could then be shared through a searchable Internet of neighborhoods across the country. As I learned from Deborah Estrin, a small-data pioneer *and* active leader in the field of public health, the technology that could one day power such an Internet is far less important than the social process to build it. As a major contributor to the development of the Internet's fundamental underlying technologies, she would know.

AN INTERNET OF NEIGHBORHOOD SMALL DATA

We are awash in small data–driven insights. Anyone who has used a navigation system in a car would be familiar with the concept: information about where you are is placed in the broader context of where you could go (a map), and you get continual feedback based upon where you want to go (a destination). In exchange for this information, services like Google Maps are able to gather the movement information from millions of people to help give you even more feedback about traffic patterns and alternative routes. This is the same information that is put together for commercial uses, by Google or Facebook for example, to drive personalized advertising. These companies learn what streams of small data mean to you, based upon how you react to it or if you ignore it entirely. They can use this information to classify behavior and choices, combine streams of data in new ways, and anticipate new services that should exist to solve common patterns of challenges or unrecognized opportunity. Despite reasonable fears about what this information is used for, Americans are sharing more, influencing each other, and being influenced by these feedback-driven insights.

Taken together, individuals or neighborhoods that exchange small data are able to do three things: (1) recognize where they are in a broader context, enabling them to identify opportunities and develop creative ways to bypass constraints ahead, (2) adjust behavior and actions on a continuous basis to achieve self-identified aims, and (3) gain insight from the experience of others within a similar context, foreshadowing scenarios they may encounter or want to avoid.

At its core, small data is a way of thinking about using information that "connects people with timely, meaningful insights (derived from big data and/or 'local' sources), organized and packaged—often visually—to be accessible, understandable and actionable for everyday tasks."[12] People are integral participants in what, how, and why information is prioritized to yield meaningful insights. For example, Google Now and the Apple Watch both use feedback to learn what the users find meaningful about their surroundings, how they schedule their day, or what they might find interesting in a nearby location. They work through a type of affirmative inquiry, where information is presented and a user either interacts with it because it is useful or simply ignores it or states that it is not useful. Over time, the service learns the basic flow of your life, no doubt with the secondary intent of selling highly contextual and relevant services and products. In a similar way, our family, social supporters, and professional colleagues learn information about each of us. They discover a lot about our habits, preferences, and decision-making process, which allows them to be influential in how we assemble our lives. This is often how someone new becomes an integral part of our lives, whether as a community health worker or a friend.

For SCALE, the exchange of insights takes place within and across a network of 20 pacesetters, which have the help of mentors and topical and regional hubs. The mentors are able to quickly appreciate what challenge a pacesetter is facing and facilitate a search for insights to help them along. What type of network would have the ability to exchange neighborhood-level insights in a country with a couple hundred thousand neighborhoods, and what could you learn from the relatively tiny network that SCALE represents?

This is exactly the sort of question that Estrin, now a professor of public health and computer science at Cornell Tech in New York City, has worked on in various ways for decades. Today she is trying to learn what *one* person could teach us about health and healthcare in an era when people generally believe that you need thousands, if not millions, of people to find patterns that might be generally useful. As a computer scientist by training, she gravitated to mobile devices, like phones, as ways to learn about what a person was doing without having to ask him or her directly. Along with co-founders Ida Sim and David Haddad, she formed Open mHealth to design "a common language for health data,"[13] regardless of where it comes from or why it exists. Given the right feedback and connectivity, people could find ways to improve their own health and help others to do the same. By analogy, how is it that one community within a neighborhood can create the conditions of a healthier life whereas another struggles? Evaluating both communities enables a neighborhood to harness its full potential. In Estrin's view, the key to improved health resides in our ability, as individuals, families, or communities, to use the information around us to assemble a better life and society. What we're missing is the right type of connectivity to share these insights.

Because Estrin came from the computer science realm, technology was her bridge to exploring how small-data approaches provide a person practical feedback to improve his or her health. For example, if a diabetic patient has information about her own blood sugar, activity, and eating patterns using a suite of sensors, she could engage in her own care in a form of "participatory sensing." More to the point, she would have knowledge of where she was with regard to her biology, diet, and exercise and could adjust accordingly. The same principle applies to a neighborhood, where a theory of change gives rise to a set of processes that help a group of people achieve a goal, and they need a method for gaining feedback along the way. When seen in tandem with 20 other neighborhoods, they form a distributed network of people and places that are searching and sensing their way to healthier lives.

Although there may never be such a high emphasis on technology in the SCALE communities, Estrin's insights encouraged SCALE's measurement team to develop a schema that prioritizes qualitative and quantitative feedback that fosters conversation at the smallest level, rather than privileging decision-makers at the top. In fact, this is what Estrin has been doing her entire career.

Estrin wrote her dissertation on intra-organizational networks in 1985 at MIT, where she also received a degree in technology policy. At the time, the effort to route communications across networks was pragmatic work that was overshadowed in prestige by developing the computing architecture that required connecting. She made seminal contributions to the early Internet before branching off even further to one of the most fringe areas: connecting other types of inputs and sensors ("simple systems"; "Internet of things") to this network. As she recalled the early days of ARPANET (the pre-Internet), I heard echoes of the task SCALE had given itself:

> You can't build an Internet by yourself. You can't by its definition, if there wasn't community agreement for what the Internet should do. The original ARPANET was created to link the small number of computer centers around the country to share resources in standard ways because, at the time, they were limited. It turned out to be the one thing that was not useful, because computing power became plentiful! Although the original motivation went away—to share a small number of computer resources—the foundation was laid in ARPANET's packet switch network. ARPANET grew into the Internet, became a conglomeration of different types of network; Ethernet on a campus connected to the backbone, using the single protocol that the world uses. A simple way of talking to computers made these networks user friendly, and ARPANET spread like wildfire. The reason the Internet worked is that there was a minimal set of requirements for global agreement. You need a really minimal parsimonious set of things that everyone has to do, and elaborate requirements don't work because it gets harder to get agreement and conformity and leaves you less nimble.[14]

Because of her seminal contributions to how computing networks operate, Estrin was asked to chair a Defense Advanced Research Policy Agency (DARPA) committee that produced a report on distributed sensors entitled *Embedded, Everywhere*, in 2001.[15] She recognized that these technologies needed an "application domain" to truly advance, and found her way to ecology before arriving in the health domain.

Estrin and her colleagues recognize they cannot build a parallel universe of technology-based sensors and devices to stream information in order to bring small data into the mainstream. Instead, they operate under the premise that people are the most sensitive and insightful "sensors" of their environment, and that other sources of information of how people interact complete the picture. She focuses on how individuals assemble their lives—movement data from smartphones, continuous TV usage, food bills, topics of concern that they search for on the Internet, peak times of social interaction—with the goal of enabling individuals and communities to see these traces for themselves. In some basic sense, she gives people an opportunity to reflect upon their actions, their traces in the world, and see how they are connected to a bigger environment. This *small data mindset* is similar to what an expert health coach would elicit in an MI session, where a person's reflections are then amplified and shaped into a narrative of action that they help create.

BRINGING SMALL DATA TO SCALE

The SCALE team embraced these principles of exchange and small data as they sought to identify measures that give neighborhoods insights about where they are improving. These measures would need to reflect change across physical, mental, social, and spiritual dimensions, overlaid upon individual/population, community, and societal levels. Many were drawn from the Institute of Medicine's *Vital Signs*, RWJF's *Culture of Health Measures*, Gallup-Healthways Well-Being Index, and other existing sources. These would allow pacesetters to focus on developing thoughtful initiatives, learn if they were making an impact, and share their process with other pacesetters.

For example, faith leaders within a pacesetter community may sponsor a contest for their respective congregations to lower their blood pressure as a collective goal. They may have come to the idea independently, or heard about it elsewhere, but they are more likely to do it successfully if they have the ability to search for best practices and exchange what they learn when they accomplish their goals. In the process of this exchange, a sharing economy for health improvement emerges, where tools and processes (new recipes, ways to build a successful contest) can be swapped and combined in novel approaches to help individuals and communities unlock their own path to improvement. Far from being disconnected from big-data sources or evidence-based policies that are common in public health and healthcare, the small-data mindset privileges our lives and neighborhood context first.

David Erickson hopes that this exchange may lead to a "quasi-market" for health. He defines three categories of actors needed to help define the parameters of a quasi-market for total population health: (1) buyers of health (population health–focused healthcare organizations, public health systems, patients, neighbors, consumers), (2) sellers of health (services focused upon "upstream" interventions like improving housing, education, or economic security), and (3) toolmakers who can facilitate the interaction (e.g., social impact bonds, management systems, technologists). "If you can get that market up and going—you won't need to coordinate that much. Outcome-based financing can solve that wrong pocket problem."[16] The outcomes he refers to are substantially better health and opportunity for individuals and families than what their neighborhood averages currently suggest. Since the modern market is embedded in a network of social interactions, Erickson and Estrin purposefully fuse ideas from economics and technology, respectively, in primary service of health improvement.

Through SCALE, the 100M Campaign learns how to create a small world of customized support, where improvement can be sparked by a neighbor, neighboring town, or a place within an intimate network and sustained through feedback, insight, and affirmation. Doing this in a way that can be guided by evidence, best practice, and recognition of the policy environment is part of the bargain. But how can large-scale networks that connect neighborhoods efficiently exchange and search for insights that apply to their context?

The success of SCALE, and the 100M Campaign more broadly, is predicated upon as many participants as possible sharing a common language and mutual understandings of how the network operates. It also depends upon fostering deeply meaningful relationships and commitment to improving the health and well-being of their neighborhoods. The dynamism of the network emerges from a pervasive pressure to continuously make sense of the raw ideas that are generated at the neighborhood level. Even once a common aim is set, it is not obvious how to ensure the "right measures" are in place to improve the quality of efforts, or that the most successful arrangements to ensure mutual accountability are well known. This last factor—mutual accountability—is possibly the most crucial, as it allows the interconnected parts of a place to more fluidly exchange the financing required to alleviate the "wrong pocket" problems that plague the country. One of the objectives of the 100M Campaign's Community Health Improvement Academy is to strategize how the right measures and the right terms of accountability can be sought.

FILLING IN THE GAPS

As organizations clumped together in joining the 100M Campaign, they began to see themselves as a COIN that provided expertise or experience in strengthening the quality of work within neighborhoods, or helping them to construct the right scaffolds so they could fill the gaps they would inevitably encounter. (Ultimately, every neighborhood, like every American, will encounter a scenario where it will need support or expertise that is not easily available.) Soma Stout calls these "topical hubs" and "capability" hubs, which function as a national-level COIN (see table 10.1). Over time, it is expected that new hubs will form as missing elements are identified, multiply as a hub topic is felt to be too big, or collapse as people realize that they are more likely to succeed together as a unified group. This organic structure is a powerful way to allow people to sit on the sidelines of an effort until they are ready to join or slow down and recruit the support they need before moving forward. For example, as news spreads that healthcare systems are obligated to perform community need assessments and spend money on community health benefits to maintain their nonprofit status, networks of nonhealthcare organizations within a neighborhood should be getting ready to articulate their aims in ways that could be fulfilled by this financing source. By simply being aware of the respective pressures and timelines on different parts of the total neighborhood-based health system, a local healthcare system may realize that it needs to slow down decision-making and instead shift to strengthening its neighborhood-based partners.

As in any large-scale process, the nature of how consensus happens reflects its most essential character and behavior (e.g., "representative democracy," "technically driven," "majority rules"). Knowing it would influence the entire 100M Campaign, the type of consensus process that SCALE chose

TABLE 10.1
Topical and Capability Hubs

Topical Hubs	Capability Hubs
Measure and close equity gaps	Shift culture and mindset
Give all kids a great start	Learn about and facilitate development of peer-to-peer support systems at the level of the block
Address the social determinants of health across the continuum	Make sustainable funding strategies accessible to a critical mass of health systems and communities
Make mental health everybody's job	Integrate data across silos to help create an integrated picture of strengths, assets, and needs
Use the top chronic diseases and core risk factors relevant to each community to build a multisectoral continuum of health and capability in behavior change	Transform primary care + healthcare financing
Help veterans thrive	Engage employers and businesses to transform the experience of work
Engage people in their own health	Build a health workforce strategy that crosses boundaries
Create the best possible well-being at the end of life	Measures that matter

"Strategic Priorities," 100 Million Healthier Lives webpage, accessed December 15, 2015, http://www.ihi.org/Engage/Initiatives/100MillionHealthierLives/Pages/Approach.aspx.

is consequential in achieving its aims. Estrin introduced one process to the campaign that has proved both successful and influential elsewhere: the model of *rough consensus* used to build the Internet.

ROUGH CONSENSUS AND RUNNING CODE

Today, the Internet's infrastructure is governed by bodies like the Internet Engineering Task Force (IETF) which work to stabilize and evolve its structure as millions of co-creators bring to light new opportunities and challenges that deserve technical attention. Since there are potentially hundreds of interests at work to define the technical parameters that inform a possible new function, ranging from commercial promise to academic inquiry to engineering requirements, the process of achieving consensus to allow for reliable norms and sufficient openness is an old challenge of governing for the public good. The IETF method is an exercise in polycentric governance over the design of the Internet, analogous to the SCALE effort to improve neighborhood health without controlling the decisions that individuals and neighborhoods collectively make.

All members of the IETF (only individuals can be members, not organizations) agree that a technically sound Internet is the first priority, just as individual members of a pacesetter community are committed to the campaign goal. In the IETF process, anything is by definition permitted unless it breaks the fundamental architecture of the Internet. In its most essential form it means that the protocols that define its hourglass structure, and those that are dependent upon it, should not be compromised. The *structure* of the Internet is constrained by the technologies that limit its bandwidth, reliability, and speed. Its fundamental *logic* is encoded in simple and universal protocols that specify how bits of information are shared (e.g., TCP/IP). This enables a nearly infinite combination of content and applications that travel across the Inter-Network (network of networks), which can be connected to any number of things that can plug in.

In the context of SCALE and the 100M Campaign, anything that reduced the intrinsic motivation of neighborhoods to improve their health or diminished the exchange of creative insights across the growing SCALE network would break its fundamental architecture and compromise the campaign's goals. Otherwise, the sky was the limit for building upon it.

There is a short but influential document that guides decision-making for the Internet, "On Consensus and Humming in the IETF," which emphasizes consensus should be *rough*. This is particularly significant where nearly all decisions can have many possible "right answers." In this sense rough consensus is the path, not the destination:

As a working group does its work and makes its choices, it behaves as if it is striving toward full consensus and tries to get all issues addressed to the satisfaction of everyone in the group, even those who originally held objections ... However, when a participant says, "That's not my favorite solution, but I can live with it; I'm satisfied that we've made a reasonable choice," that participant is not in the "rough" part of a rough consensus; the group actually reached consensus if that person is satisfied with the outcome. It's when the chair has to declare that an unsatisfied person still has an open issue, but that the group has truly answered the objection, that the consensus is only rough. [17]

When facing a "wicked problem" like building a healthier neighborhood, for example, adopting rough consensus does not require that severe constraints be placed upon decision-making. For example, there is no need to state that the only way forward for improving population health in a neighborhood is if actions are evidence based or value based. These are certainly important standards, and should be included in a set of approaches, but they are not the only ones. Moreover, enforcing them immediately locks out any party that is not skilled enough or traditionally conceived of as a participant, as would be the case in determining eligibility for CMMI's accountable health communities if it is ever broadly released. Allowing for rough consensus means that dissent need not be suppressed, and the potential for innovative ways of doing things remains intact. The IETF's motto, "Rough consensus and running code," fuses two important concepts. Running code means not just talking about ideas, but actually making something, testing it, and improving as you go. This concept is crucial and central to the culture of co-creation, of building new capabilities and infrastructure, of solving large-scale challenges by inventing entirely new processes to solve collective problems. Without it, "rough consensus" devolves into committees and standard-making bodies that become sclerotic and out of touch with what innovators are doing and what users actually need.

Interestingly, the IETF report only cites four sources, and one of them—a book called *Beyond Majority Rules: Voteless Decisions in the Religious Society of Friends*—may come as a surprise in a seminal document on how engineers come to consensus about the current state and future of the Internet. It describes the process by which Quaker communities make group-centered decisions, emphasizing reflection and deepened understanding of issues, where "cheap talk" is maintained until rough consensus naturally emerges.

Given the decidedly predigital inspiration for the process that the IETF uses, it is possible to see the routes to neighborhood healthcare in a new light. The Dallas town halls that PCCI used to develop consensus on what their software should accomplish for the people who attended; ISAIAH's recognition of when an issue was ready for an "action"; City Health Works's role in building higher-quality connectivity across a scattered neighborhood; or CHA's radical engagement of its staff and patient community to redesign healthcare all point to discovering some principles of polycentric governance, collaborative networks, or ways to achieve consensus. None of the organizations discussed in part 2, however, had the benefit of foresight that the Community Health Improvement Academy could provide: how to create a successful COIN, methods of building and achieving consensus, how to improve the quality of processes or the accountability of partners, and methods of sustaining financing for initiatives that span many organizations or sectors. Nor has the Academy yet had the opportunity to absorb their methods and spread them across the network. For now, at least, SCALE remains a small part of the larger 100M Campaign, which continues to grow at a brisk pace with hundreds of member organizations joining each quarter.

A HARLEM HUB

When I heard that SCALE would be searching for pacesetters, I finally felt that my journey would translate into something useful for living a healthier life in Harlem. After Ray's death, I sought out the advice of Harlem-based organizations that were making a difference in the lives of people like him, his daughter, and his grandchildren.

Since Ray had struggled to find a job after coming back from Vietnam, I gravitated toward an organization called Strive International, which provides workforce development and job retraining, including for people who have been incarcerated. I was welcomed by its co-founder, Rob Carmona, who has spent decades building Strive from a local organization to a national and international model. Carmona seemed to know everyone in the neighborhood. For Strive to do its job, it has to make and maintain high-quality connections with nonprofits, social service agencies, and businesses that could offer jobs to the alumni of its programs. The organization's leaders quickly recognized that although they had a reputation in the labor sector, the opportunities that their alumni had enjoyed led to transformations in not only their health, but also the health of their family. When Carmona heard about SCALE, he immediately reached out to colleagues at the Harlem Children's Zone, City Health Works, the Mount Sinai Health System, and a few others. Together, they developed an application that conveyed their vision of what they wanted to accomplish together that could not be done alone. Although some of Carmona's colleagues were initially skeptical that their workforce organization could be a leading force in health improvement, the process of thinking through how these organizations could work together and leverage their neighborhood networks won them over.

When the finalist mentor and pacesetter communities were announced in Grapevine, Texas, I was disappointed that my colleagues in Harlem had not been chosen.[18] On the other hand, a close look at the communities that did make the cut was both inspiring and instructive (see box 10.2). As I headed home from the conference where the SCALE selections had been announced, I was heartened to get a note from Carmona. His words reflected the sentiment of the Harlem group: "We want to see about moving forward like we WERE selected."

When I read his note, I thought about Ray, my first few months of residency, and how much I had learned by meeting people who helped me understand why it was nearly impossible to assemble a healthier life in Harlem without having the right pieces at our fingertips, both as a neighbor or a healthcare professional. Now, after four years, I had met a group of dedicated people and organizations that were invested in working together to build a neighborhood-based health system.

Since I was by then intimately familiar with the 100M Campaign and the precepts of SCALE, I felt that our Harlem group could learn some of the basics that the pacesetters would be learning through the Academy. This would enable the group to work together, draw other neighborhood groups in, and maintain a sense of mutual accountability in the process. As I saw the neighborhood from the inside out, it was clear that the gap between certain neighborhood organizations was substantial and deeply consequential. As motivated as the Harlem group was, its members had minimal interaction with one another and with the large healthcare systems within and around the neighborhood—including one of its co-applicants, Mount

Sinai Health System! With the exception of Mount Sinai, none of these organizations were recognized as part of the city's public health system, so they were obviously not benefitting from its experience and expertise. They were only dimly aware of the collective impact models that some leading community development organizations were looking to advance through support of groups just like them.

To be effective, Carmona's Harlem group needed to develop awareness of other organizations that served the same people, as well as the healthcare and public health systems that play an outsized role in the work of shaping the terms of what health improvement entails.

BOX 10.2
Selection of Pacesetters Chosen for SCALE Initiative

Algoma, WI
- Live Algoma Coalition
- Bellin Health
- School District of Algoma
- Precision Machine Inc.

Atlanta, GA
- Atlanta Regional Collaborative for Health Improvement (ARCHI)
- Georgia State University Research Foundation's Georgia Health Policy Center
- Atlanta Regional Commission
- United Way of Greater Atlanta
- St. Joseph's Mercy Care
- Kaiser Permanente
- Grady Health System

Cattaraugus County, NY
- Cattaraugus County Health Department
- Cattaraugus County Department of Aging

- Healthy Community Alliance
- Southern Tier Health Care System
- Salamanca Youth Center
- University Primary Care

Hennepin County, MN
- Hennepin Health Foundation, Hennepin Healthcare System, Inc. d/b/a Hennepin County Medical Center (HCMC)
- Hennepin County Human Services and Public Health Department, Public Health Promotion
- Northwest Hennepin Family Services Collaborative
- North Sky Health Consulting
- Brooklyn Park, Minnesota

Laramie County, WY
- Laramie County Community Partnership, Inc.
- HealthWorks
- Cheyenne Regional Medical Center

- United Way of Laramie County
- Laramie County Community College

Maricopa County, AZ
- Maricopa County Department of Public Health
- Maricopa County Community College District (MCCCD)
- Banner Health
- Esperança
- City of Phoenix-FitPHX

North Colorado
- North Colorado Health Alliance
- Weld County Department of Public Health and Environment
- Sunrise Community Health (FQHC)
- United Way of Weld County
- High Plains Library District

Salt Lake City, UT
- Ethnic Community-based Organization for Refugees
- Musungu HIV/AIDS Support Organization
- Burundi Drummers
- The Church of Jesus Christ of Latter-day Saints (Community Outreach Division)

San Francisco, CA
- Saint Francis Foundation
- Saint Francis Memorial Hospital
- San Francisco Department of Public Health
- San Francisco Mayor's Office of Economic and Workforce Development
- University of California San Francisco
- Boys and Girls Clubs of San Francisco

San Gabriel Valley, CA
- City of Hope
- Neighbors Acting Together Helping All (NATHA)
- City of Duarte
- Duarte Unified School District (DUSD)

Sitka, AK
- Sitka Health Summit
- Southeast Alaska Regional Hospital Consortium
- Sitka Community Hospital
- Braveheart Volunteers

Waterville, ME
- Healthy Northern Kennebec
- Kennebec Behavioral Health
- Kennebec Valley Community Action Program
- Waterville Main Street
- Family Violence Project
- City of Waterville

Press Release, "IHI Announces Final Selection of Communities for Health-Focused SCALE Initiative," April 17, 2015, http://www.ihi.org/about/news/Documents/IHIPress-Release_IHIAnnouncesSCALEAwardees_Apr15.pdf

11

Integrating the Whole

*It takes a while to learn how to use an entirely new system
and reconfigure practices to benefit from it.*
—David Cutler, *The Quality Cure*

DESIGNING WITH THE END IN MIND

One of the motivations for the Harlem group's application to SCALE was the opportunity to access the considerable finances "locked in" the healthcare sector. They hoped that by having their collective contribution "count" toward the value proposition of improved total population health, they could share in its financing. But for now, even relatively well-developed systems that are important for a healthier life, like education or transportation, have low or no connectivity to healthcare systems and the considerable money "locked in" the healthcare sector, leaving financing that may be best spent out of healthcare's pocket stuck and used in a less impactful way. As these connections are forged, the language and infrastructures needed to allow them to flourish will have to be constructed.

In 1994, a trio of scholars who were originally trained in economics, and subsequently branched into the management, politics, and policy of healthcare, edited an influential volume entitled *Why Are Some People Healthy and Others Are Not?* In it, they persuasively conveyed that no one entity is *functionally* responsible for the health of the total population in a place:

> Precision is gained at a cost. Narrow definitions leave out less specific dimensions of health that many people would judge to be important to their evaluation of their own circumstances, or those of their associates. On the other hand, it seems at least plausible that the broad range of determinants of health

whose effects are reflected in the "mere absence of disease or injury," or simple survival, is also relevant to more comprehensive definitions of health. [1]

The authors then attempted to build an analytic framework, "component by component, progressively adding complexity," to allow readers to become more aware of how healthcare systems are conceived, and how the definitions of health within those systems are often static and incomplete. They describe the necessity of building a healthcare system that is capable of more varied and complex interactions—not only with the people it serves, but also with the places where they live. In 2002, David Kindig of the University of Wisconsin and Greg Stoddart of McMaster University (a co-author of the passage on precision) built upon this work in "What Is Population Health?" They define it as "the health outcomes of individuals, including the distribution of such outcomes within the group."[2] This language, which differs from public health definitions of health through its focus on individuals, and from healthcare definitions of health because of its focus on equitable health outcomes of a group, began to flood the space that traditionally separates healthcare and public health. The scholars then sought professionals or practitioners, citizens or consumers, who identified with this definition of population health.

By 2012, there was considerable momentum building around population health, and Dawn Jacobson and Steven Teutsch looked at how the term was being used in practice, which they defined in a working paper for the National Quality Forum.[3] From their work, they defined "total population health" as all the people in a geopolitical area—in contrast to subpopulations, such as a group of insured patients. In their framework, they saw the work of improving total population health as requiring a "system-within-a-system," where healthcare systems, education systems, employer systems, for example, represent subsystems with their own populations that contribute to the *total* population.[4]

Their definition, which reflects how neighborhoods, with or without success, *functionally* work to improve total population health, is precisely what the Accountable Health Communities initiative aimed to bring to healthcare systems. In its prerelease incarnation, the CMMI model would begin by making healthcare systems more aware of the assets in their neighborhoods that contribute to total population health. Then it aimed to progressively support the creation of navigation pathways and community health hubs that are similar to what Mark and Sarah Redding have pioneered in Ohio. Since all CMMI models are fundamentally about changing how healthcare is financed, Darshak Sanghavi knew that his ability to release it depended upon how well his group would be able to measure and attribute better health outcomes and quality at lower cost to the CMMI model.[5] The Accountable Health Community effort is predicated upon achieving progressively higher levels of systemic awareness for what neighborhoods need to do to improve total population health. In turn, this awareness should translate into better health outcomes, higher-quality connections between mutually accountable partners, and lower overall healthcare costs. It represents an evolutionary step in the development of healthcare systems that see their primary role as contributing to total population health.

SYSTEMIC AWARENESS

In some sense, criticism about a local healthcare system's inability to think outside of its own box often stems from the density of activity within its own walls and networks and the relative inability of organizations that contribute to health in the neighborhood—transportation, education, social agencies, and neighborhood organizations—to coherently interact with it. Put another way, healthcare organizations are too inwardly focused, and everyone else in the neighborhood finds them too complicated and distractible to co-create the best pathways to total population health.

To its credit, the healthcare sector has developed self-evaluative processes at nearly every level that enable large networks of activity to prioritize effort according to internally defined aims and measures. These self-evaluative processes—developing quality requirements, discovering and defining modes of accountability, and sustaining cycles of financial investment—result in self-contained, sectorwide behavior that makes an individual hospital or healthcare system seem impenetrably complex from the outside looking in. The totality of these processes reinforces feedback loops for reinvestment, error correction, and adaptation. However, it is too easy for regional healthcare systems to lose touch with what it takes for people to live healthier lives within their immediate geographic context, where regional populations are likely to be rooted for generations to come.[6]

With guidance, healthcare systems that are financially accountable for the health of neighborhood populations can adjust their priorities accordingly. There are three key areas where healthcare would benefit from investing in the capability of public health systems and the community development industry to share its system attributes: (1) *quality requirements*: the ability to generate and share information about the de facto structure of the neighborhood public health system, processes that cross boundaries within neighborhoods, and how they influence total population health outcomes; (2) *accountability*: the ability to clearly define boundaries of culpability and lines of responsibility with an emphasis on neighbors as "citizen-members" of a place; and (3) *financial sustainability*: the ability to clearly articulate how a short- or medium-term process or function adds value to a long-term pathway of improved total population health.

It is important to understand how these system properties—quality, accountability, and financial sustainability—drive healthcare system improvement, and how these same properties create opportunities for connectivity between public health systems and community development. In composite, we arrive at neighborhood-based systems for improving total population health. As neighborhood-based systems integrate with 100M Campaign networks at the regional and national level, unprecedented opportunities to redesign healthcare systems emerge.

HOW AMERICA'S HEALTHCARE SYSTEM ARCHITECTS ITSELF

Quality Requirements

For nearly four decades, the Institute of Medicine has released a series of influential and authoritative reports on quality, safety, measurability, and improvability of various aspects of the American healthcare system. These adjectives are termed "-ilities"; they allow someone to judge how a system is operating, as opposed to simply focusing upon what it is doing. For instance, improving the *quality* in healthcare has been a consistent theme over the past three decades (a central focus for national integrators like the IOM and IHI), and the diverse perspectives on quality (practitioners, patients, academics, policy makers) have given healthcare multiple interconnected views of the same property. In the language of systems, -ilities are *nonfunctional requirements* that help define its architecture (e.g., *accessibility* describes a healthcare system principle), as opposed to the *functional requirements* that define its design (e.g., a nurse should be able to triage X number of patients to the right level of care in an hour). Interestingly, all nonfunctional requirements put together describe a system's *quality re-quirements*, which is why the concept echoes at multiple levels of healthcare. The -ilities can be further subdivided into being execution-oriented, which can be observed as they happen (e.g., usability), or evolution-oriented, which are embodied by overarching behaviors (e.g., sustainability). These attributes can be rephrased into more familiar language: "Is a healthcare system patient-centered?"—which is execution-oriented; and, "Does the healthcare system make the right investments over time?"—which is evolution-oriented.

The rationale for investment, innovation, and improvement follows the development of quality requirements in a self-reinforcing way. When the Institute of Medicine released the landmark report *To Err Is Human*[7] in 1999, patient-advocacy groups, the public, physicians, healthcare administrators, and purchasers of services shifted their attention to address patient safety in the hospital. Fortunately, leaders in quality improvement, who frequently convene at the IOM, have provided clear direction on how to establish quality measures that can apply to any organization or entity that plays a role in improving health.[8] In a *Journal of the American Medical Association* article entitled "What Makes a Good Quality Measure?" the authors state: "The first step is to determine whether a particular process should be related to a particular outcome . . . The second step, if evidence exists to establish an expected process-outcome relationship, is to determine the magnitude of that relationship . . . The third step is to consider the difference in outcomes that might be reasonable to expect with optimal performance on the measure being evaluated."[9]

In these terms, a useful quality measure could be, for example, whether appropriate precautions had been taken to prevent an infection from all of the needles and IV lines that are routinely inserted into patients during their hospital stay. The first step is establishing that infections can occur from improperly inserted IV lines. The second step is to know how a hospital's infection rate stacks up to the industry standard, which depends upon the site of the IV, and then the third is to know if differences from the standard are significant, particularly in specific cases.

Because the exact causes of Ray's rapid deterioration and death were not fully known, I presented his case in a full-quality review (called M&Ms for Morbidity and Mortality Rounds). Although a quality-improvement officer continuously reviews individual patient cases, the M&M in my department was held on a nearly monthly basis, where a resident like myself either volunteered a patient case he or she thought had had a poor outcome, or was assigned one to investigate.

The M&M, which is a historic institution in medicine, represents a formal forum to reflect upon social and cultural factors that influence the quality of systems of care. Every physician who was involved in the care of the patient attends, including, in Ray's case, the pathologist who allowed me to observe his autopsy. Together, the entire room of physicians notes opportunities for improvement, often at crucial moments where the workflows of different teams intersect, where joint decision-making is required, or, perhaps, where an intimidating context may have interfered with seeking appropriate help.

At the time, I already knew why Ray's case had been brought to the fore: he had acquired an IV-related hospital infection, likely from a line that remained in too long amidst the shuffle from the hospital floor to the ICU. I presented Ray's case in early 2012, at a time when hospitals were placing intensive focus on reducing the number of IV line insertion–related bloodstream infections to zero, a measure that provided focus for a patient safety movement, backed by the stick of losing financial payments for an entire hospital stay if this occurred.

My role at the M&M was to present a rigorous review of the data, timelines, and context of the case, as well as to provide insight into my decision-making along the way, enriched with the benefit of hindsight. I did not have an iota of concern about a punitive response for making a mistake, aside from my own sense of responsibility to exhaustively illuminate my role in the context of a broader system. However, we did find many opportunities for improvement in his care, including further inquiry over the appropriate level of staffing for a holiday weekend.

Across the nation, healthcare systems invested in patient safety techniques and quality improvement methods, which also shone a spotlight on the team-based nature of preventing errors. Healthcare quality measures are increasingly publicly available and poor quality motivates a redesign of how entire processes of care take place. Consequently, *quality requirements* as a systemic property create a rationale for healthcare systems to look within and beyond their current state of operation. Quality is intimately linked to accountability.

Accountability

In chapter 10, I introduced Elinor Ostrom's rules for the structure of mutual accountability in systems of polycentric governance. Unfortunately, references to accountability for health are as pervasive as a consistent definition is elusive. In a 1999 document with a title that conveys its motivation— "Accountability—The Pathway for Restoring Public Trust and Confidence for Hospitals and Other Health Care Organizations"[10]—the American Hospital Association tried to articulate what the term meant for its own members. They assembled a range of definitions, including one from Larry Gamm that frames accountability in terms of the quality requirements of a system: "Accountability of health services organizations is defined as taking into account and responding to political, commercial, community, and clinical/patient interests and expectations. Accountability is the process by which health leaders pursue the objectives of efficiency, quality, and access to meet the interests and expectations of these significant 'publics.'"[11]

This immediately brings into question who or what constitutes the "publics," which future contributors to the ACA, Ezekiel Emmanuel and his colleague Linda Emmanuel, answered by stating that there are "different parties [who] should be held accountable or hold others accountable." They went on to elaborate that there are three models of accountability:

> We characterize and compare three dominant models of accountability:
> 1) the professional model, in which the individual physician and patient
> participate in shared decision making and physicians are held accountable
> to professional colleagues and to patients; 2) the economic model, in which
> the market is brought to bear in health care and accountability is mediated
> through consumer choice of providers; and 3) the political model, in which
> physicians and *patients interact as citizen-members within a community* and
> in which physicians are accountable to a governing board elected from the
> members of the community, such as the board of a managed care plan.[12]
> [my emphasis]

The first two are well developed, where a physician and patient are accountable to each other, and the "market is brought to bear in health care and accountability is mediated through consumer choice of providers," respectively. The third, the political model, is less familiar to healthcare. This type might presage a future definition of accountability in population health, but for the fact that Emanuel's example of the governing board is "the board of a managed care plan." Obviously, healthcare's political accountability is more intimately tied to a feedback loop of economic interests than to a place-based, democratically governed "community." Even though the ACO model extends the territory of the healthcare system's interest to a patient's daily life decisions in the neighborhood (e.g., diabetes lifestyle management), the development of effective engagement systems that fit this new context remains anemic. Healthcare investors (both public and private) continue to search for high-leverage, minimalist strategies that convert the neighborhood context into a more controlled environment for consumer-oriented patient care, answerable to the economic and political interests that aren't necessarily aligned with those of the neighborhood.

Financial Sustainability

How healthcare systems are financed is an enduring and historic driver of healthcare system architecture *and* design. Even public hospitals, like New York City's Health and Hospitals Corporation (HHC) led by Ram Raju, make their financing strategy a priority, just as the privately held Hospital Corporation of America (HCA) does. Today, the rising costs of care for patients fundamentally shapes how healthcare systems are architected, which is the ultimate concession of an expert-driven sector to the political and economic reality of its largesse. The irony is that a concession to consumers, for example, strengthens healthcare's power and influence: it appears that despite the theoretical role of consumers in keeping healthcare costs low, drug prices, insurance premiums, and overall healthcare costs are projected to rise, which simply shifts the potential savings of healthcare reform to other parts of the healthcare sector.[13] For a neighborhood of citizen-members to be a relevant force in defining the aims of healthcare systems, we need to know the costs of care at the total population level (an Institute of Medicine [IOM] Vital Sign). Then we need to know significantly more about the factors that affect it in the short (1 year) and medium (3–5 years) term, which are relevant time frames to influence and synchronize the decision-making of healthcare and public health systems, as well as community development efforts in the neighborhood.

However, to truly take advantage of the perspectives of citizen-members in the neighborhood, the political and economic risks of ignoring their perspective—in terms of lost opportunities to reduce total population costs of care and diminished political support—must be made clear. Some health-care systems are trying to integrate the citizen-member view into their financing and operational logic. Take the ACA's new IRS reporting require-ment for nonprofit healthcare systems to demonstrate community benefit in order to maintain their tax-exempt status. As noted in part one, many hospital administrators consider this a box to be checked for providing uncompensated care for the uninsured, an option that is receding in states that have expanded Medicaid coverage. As monies for community bene-fit become more available because more healthcare insurance coverage means that fewer dollars can be chalked up to "uncompensated care," will they be reabsorbed into existing functions, or thoughtfully invested for the long-term benefit of the neighborhoods where the healthcare system's sub-populations reside? Some systems, like Kaiser Permanente on the West Coast, have definitively chosen the latter. Their work is led by Tyler Norris, one of 100M's chief organizers, in his role as vice president of Total Health Partnerships, where he shares Kaiser Permanente's belief that the organiza-tion will be around for the long haul, for its patients, employees, and their neighborhoods:

> To affect measurable population level behavior and health changes, you
> can't make a grant, and then expect lasting change in just two or three years.
> We take a longer view, focusing on community assets and environments,
> and help build the long-term capacity of community partners. The latter is
> vital so that communities build the collective efficacy that is requisite to ef-
> fecting measurable impact, at scale, with sufficient reach and intensity, over
> time. The stronger community bonds and assets we help forge, the better
> our clinical offerings can integrate with community supports in a way that
> assures total health and well-being.[14]

In practical terms, this means that Kaiser Permanente's community benefit fund, which amounts to over $1 billion, can be reinvested in creative and necessary partnerships that lead to better health in the neighborhoods where their beneficiaries and employees live. Kaiser Permanente's leader-ship hired Norris to develop sustained, structurally important partnerships with neighborhood organizations and employer unions. When I saw him in action as one of the leaders of the 100M Healthier Lives Campaign, I saw the powerful combination of his skills at work. With degrees in business and divinity as well as substantial organizing experience, he could simultaneously speak to the value of being connected, the transcendent purpose of durable coalitions, and why collective leadership is paramount at this particular moment. To proceed in creating partnerships that promote "total population health," Norris and his colleagues must design a relationship structure that builds upon the strengths of Kaiser Permanente's partners while gaining skills in managing and utilizing community benefit dollars effectively. It is significant that Kaiser Permanente has the financial size and principled commitment to supporting Norris's intra-preneurial activity. For those healthcare systems that do not yet have all the ingredients to embrace and act upon the total population health perspective, a *system* of public health—as opposed to a government office of public health—must emerge to form a sustainable bridge between healthcare and its citizen-members.

BUILDING SYSTEMS FOR TOTAL POPULATION HEALTH

My public health colleagues in New York City, unlike their counterparts in the larger healthcare picture, rarely talk about their own quality requirements. Absent from the public health discourse is discussion of the quality of connections between programs and within them, or about the quality of the overarching system that designs and tests these programs. Slowly but surely, pioneers in public health are working to change that.

In her work at the Department of Health and Human Services, Peggy Honoré is on a mission to bring quality to the center of public health discussions:

> When you talk about the "quality" of drinking water, you think about the characteristics that describe it: color, taste, and smell. Same with clinical patient care—patient-centered, safe, timely, and equitable, for example. Prior to the work that we started eight years ago, there were no characteristics to describe quality in public health. Instead, everyone claims, we are developing a "high quality program," but if you're not measuring that against some characteristic or standard, then it's not really quality. As a result, there is no way you can measure quality in the public health system domestically or cross nationally.[15]

Honoré learned the importance of this discussion soon after she finished her doctorate in healthcare administration and began her first assignment as chief financial officer of a state health department with a large budget:

> I naturally looked for those things in public health that I was trained to do in finance and healthcare: Where is the finance professional organization for public health? Where is the academic training in finance to help a public health organization achieve goals on its own terms? There was none. Where was the focus on quality and educational training on quality? There was none. Because it was a new environment, because I had this training in other industries, I immediately found these gaps. It has been a challenge to address those gaps because it requires bringing in something new, which some leaders distrust or do not understand.

Honoré was not simply expressing a healthcare bias in a public health context. She has a remarkably diverse professional background, starting with a finance career with Exxon and McDonald's, to senior roles in healthcare organizations, to the financial and academic officer for two state health departments. She is also the AmeriHealth Mercy-General Russel Honoré[16] Endowed Professor at Louisana State University, lent by LSU to the government for nearly a decade for her broadly recognized work to refine the concept of quality in public health. (It was for this work that she was recognized by the APHA in 2013.) Her disappointment in the direction of health and healthcare under Governor Jindal motivated her to spend time at HHS, where she hoped to pursue work that would have an impact in her home state. This makes her comfortable in a range of worlds, from healthcare system boardrooms and public health organizations to the pugnacious politics of state budgeting, all while pushing forward a grounded perspective of health improvement.

Honoré spends a significant amount of time working with public health professionals like Boston-based Catarina Hill, who is working to improve the quality of a network of mobile clinics across the nation. As Honoré interacts across a diversity of public health programs, she sees opportunities where the language and measurement of quality may drive systemic improvement in public health practice. This is in large part why the HHS's 2008 "Consensus Statement on Quality in the Public Health System" features nine characteristics of quality that together create a reference point for entities that do not traditionally see their contributions in classic health terms, even as they should logically—and functionally—be considered an essential part of the public health system (see box 11.1).[17]

BOX 11.1
Nine Characteristics of Quality in Public Health

Population-centered—protecting and promoting healthy conditions and the health for the entire population

Equitable—working to achieve health equity

Proactive—formulating policies and sustainable practices in a timely manner, while mobilizing rapidly to address new and emerging threats and vulnerabilities

Health-promoting—ensuring policies and strategies that advance safe practices by providers and the population and increase the probability of positive health behaviors and outcomes

Risk-reducing—diminishing adverse environmental and social events by implementing policies and strategies to reduce the probability of preventable injuries and illness or other negative outcomes

Vigilant—intensifying practices and enacting policies to support enhancements to surveillance activities (e.g., technology, standardization, systems thinking/modeling)

Transparent—ensuring openness in the delivery of services and practices with particular emphasis on valid, reliable, accessible, timely, and meaningful data that is readily available to stakeholders, including the public

Effective—justifying investments by utilizing evidence, science, and best practices to achieve optimal results in areas of greatest need

Efficient—understanding costs and benefits of public health interventions and to facilitate the optimal utilization of resources to achieve desired outcomes

Peggy Honoré, "Consensus Statement on Quality in the Public Health System," Health and Human Services Report, August 2008, webpage accessed December 15, 2015, http://www.hhs.gov/ash/initiatives/quality/quality/phqf-consensus-statement.html.

The importance of defining quality requirements for public health systems cannot be overstated, even if the specifics of these requirements change. Some quality characteristics, like being "proactive," can easily be applied to organizations that are not traditionally associated with health improvement—entities like schools, local businesses, and places of worship—which can then be assessed according to the same quality standards as if they were public health organizations. For example, if churches in nearby neighborhoods developed a program to support the parents of obese children in their congregation, they could assess how *proactive* their efforts were by co-creating quality measures with a local public health department or healthcare system that shares this quality requirement. When a significant network of organizations adopts the same quality measures, the likelihood that they will be calibrated and meaningfully linked to each other improves, as does the likelihood the network will expand. The same systems that measure proactivity of peer support within a church could then be used to discern how effectively elderly residents in a housing complex are updating an ailing neighbor's family. As a consequence, it becomes possible to imagine a public health professional with skills in designing proactive systems, a desirable quality that could unite unrelated sectors.

Honoré's early work at HHS was prescient, and her focus on *quality* illuminated the connection between healthcare and public health within the department:

> It was very refreshing when the ACA came out with such a heavy focus on population health. An introductory clause, "quality is a catalyst for improving population health," sits at the heart of the ACA. It is in fact a transformational quality driver to shift a nearly exclusive focus on individuals to the more critical task of need based, locally specific measures. We were focused on this before ACA, but after ACA, it really took off and more people across the department began to embrace this concept. Initially, it was very difficult. Some people [at HHS] didn't even know what public health was, that's how healthcare focused it was! That has definitely changed.

Her work also addressed the growing concern among healthcare and public health professionals that the proliferation of thousands of locally specific measures made improving public health system quality nationwide difficult to undertake. The 2011 IOM report, "America's Health in Transition:

Protecting and Improving Quality," states "there currently is no coordinated, standard set of true measures of a community's health—not aggregated information about the health of individuals residing in a community, but rather measures of green space, availability of healthy foods, land use and zoning practices that are supportive of health, safety, social capital, and social cohesion, among many other determinants of health."[18]

ASSESSING THE SYSTEM

In a system without walls, how can "aggregated information about the health of individuals residing in a community" be measured, much less assessed? As Honoré states, "Whom do you hold responsible for the health of a *population*? If infant mortality in Miami Dade is the same as a developing nation, and 2.5 times the US average rate, whom do you hold accountable for that? If your patient [Ray] died prematurely in part because of neighborhood factors, who should his daughter speak with to improve what system?"

Although the constituency of a city public health department is definitely the city's population, the department does not have the authority or capability to claim political accountability for all the neighborhood factors that affect its constituents' health. For example, even though there are 22 drug treatment programs in East Harlem that collectively cause public safety concerns, the New York City Department of Public Health does not claim accountability for resolving this issue even though these programs adversely affect the health of East Harlem residents.[19] It is a complicated matter: there may be a conflict of interest between aspects of health for one population over another; such conflicts are rarely adjudicated or even prioritized by public health professionals. And yet, by not continually striving for a political model of accountability to citizen-members, by not taking on and diffusing the political risk of making difficult decisions on a regular basis, the public health department's authority systemically diminishes. This is an example of a negative feedback loop.

A healthcare system's population, on the other hand, is the body of people who walk through its doors or are financially attributed to it. The terms of accountability in healthcare have become specific enough to be adjusted to match the needs and demands of its constituents; shortcomings within established territory are swiftly surfaced and adjudicated. This is also why moving out of a healthcare facility into the neighborhood is challenging; there is little precedent for managing the political risk of action or inaction. A public health office usually cannot enforce comprehensive policies within its geographical boundaries in the same way that hospitals can within their confines. Although this may seem obvious, the healthcare model of enforcing guidelines or protocols in a controlled environment is the one most used for public health policies and interventions. Even though it occasionally works, it simply echoes the assumptions encoded in how healthcare systems currently engage patients, rather than offering a unique public health perspective.

If public health quality requirements and accountability models are clarified, healthcare will have a reliable partner in improving total population health, and one that is ideally positioned to organize and represent citizen-members in their neighborhood as a more coherent total population health system emerges. Moreover, healthcare will learn from the substantially different operating principles and interests of public health systems, which claim to connect with other systems, like education, that influence the health of the neighborhood. Ultimately, the glue to hold this whole system together will come from incorporating direct modes of accountability to the citizen-members of the population.

In the current paradigm, public health's political accountability, like that in healthcare, is yoked to its economic model: alignment with political leadership who can requisition funds has priority over my neighbor's collective aims. This accountability model regularly generates conflict with the very same public that public health interventions are designed to benefit. Since public health departments lack both strong quality requirements and models of accountability, their conflicts with the public are nearly always seen as time for damage control rather than as opportunities for systematic improvement. Public health rarely benefits from the kinds of reinvestment cycles that make the healthcare sector more and more powerful: in public health, the quality requirements and functional requirements of the system's architecture are never stabilized because they are rarely defined in the first place.

What would it take to invest in a feedback loop governed by citizen-members with the primary aim of improving total population health? The citizen-members would have ideas not only for what would help them improve their own health, but also for how to redefine healthcare systems to help them do it. Organizations like ISAIAH and City Health Works are pioneers in this new approach, as are policy makers like Darshak Sanghavi, who aim to redefine the locus of healthcare accountability to a bounded geographical area. When I heard Sanghavi describe the Accountable Health Community at an early stage, it was clear that the boundary of a geographical site had to be flexible enough to accommodate the diverse ways in which a healthcare system may shape its own political model of accountability (e.g., neighborhood, county, region, town). In this new zone of accountability, Sanghavi envisions that a healthcare system would become aware of what a neighborhood has to offer its patients, as well as develop a newfound recognition of its critical dependencies on community groups and organizations within it, just as Parkland and PCCI are doing in Dallas. In the AHC context, the value of high-quality neighborhood connectivity emerges with a healthcare system's growing awareness of its accountability to patients as citizen-members of a place, as opposed to subpopulations that comprise an ACO (e.g., Medicare patients).

A new generation of public health systems requires public investment leveraged from three sources: (1) healthcare investments from areas that overlap with core public health priorities (early childhood development, behavioral health, healthy aging); (2) community development industry adoption of public health system quality requirements in neighborhood-level initiatives; and (3) dedicated public financing for a public health systems roadmap that drives coordinated activity at the neighborhood level ("geographic site," in AHC language) to improve total population health. Just as vital to such systems are two additional political requirements: a clear focus on citizen-members as the locus of political accountability for public health systems; and a colloquial language for total population health that my neighbors can comprehend, employ, and improve upon.

If we think back to the Healthy Bodega Initiative, it was designed in the "intervention" model of public health programming: evidence-based, expert-designed, and blessed by leadership. If it had been part of a well-defined public health system, there would have been a clear financial and operational analysis of what NYC's healthcare systems currently offered and where they might be willing to co-invest; community development financing institutions would have been enlisted to leverage their portfolio of investments in neighborhood organizations to align with the Healthy Bodega Initiative's aims; and, most importantly, the program would have been regularly iterated with the input of my neighbors, to whom the program would have been considered directly accountable. After all, any outcome that relies upon my neighbors' collective behavior change necessitates that they be given a significant hand in defining the program's usability (e.g., Is it population-centered?). Moreover, if neighborhood-based organizations like City Health Works or a public school are to be considered an integral partner in achieving a public health system's aim, their quality requirements, model of accountability, and financially sustainable contributions to a shared goal need to be equally well defined.

NEIGHBORHOOD AS A CHANNEL

Honoré considers a growing shared awareness of how neighborhood activities contribute to, or detract from, a public health system, as a priority:

> Public health will tell you it is a system, a network of organizations that intervenes at the population level to improve health. Aside from committed practitioners, all the other people—like healthcare systems, education, community development—say "we're not part of a public health system!" So it's a steep hill to climb when you want to engage people in a system of improving health that they don't even know they are a part of.

As I've explored throughout this book, the truth is that even if both healthcare and public health were able to trot out well-defined system components in a shared effort to improve a neighborhood's total population health, they would still come up short. A neighborhood is too dense with overlapping and invisible activity to account for its behavior in pre-defined terms. In fact, the apparent scatter of uncoordinated activity at the neighborhood level, shaped by how my neighbors—its citizen-members—interact with and access many different formal and informal systems, is the most compelling reason to focus on the neighborhood. Any set of solutions that are primarily driven by healthcare and public health systems will necessarily fail as the neighborhood undergoing intervention inevitably shifts its internal logic. These shifts may occur because of regional or national changes in the quality of or investment in public education, shifts in popular aesthetics for how services should be designed and delivered by other consumer industries, growing social awareness of rising costs of healthcare as health improvement stagnates, and alternative sources of healthcare that incorporate spiritual or mental dimensions more effectively. The reasons are myriad, but the outcome is the same: improvements in total population health systems are unimpressive; the underlying reasons are too complex to describe using accepted methods; political pressure for healthcare systems to reform grows as economic accountability shifts to them from insurers. Without the appropriate connectivity between neighborhood systems, and across scales of communication, we fail without insight.

To remedy this persistent failure, healthcare system transformation should be defined by the rate and capacity of the neighborhood, as the primary infrastructure for a total population health system, to become aware of its assets and relationships. A public health system anchored in this context accelerates and guides this process for all of the systems-within-systems that Jacobson and Teutsch described, particularly where multiple healthcare systems serve the same place. Instead of a place for interventions, the neighborhood is a channel for sustained, total population health improvement.

Viewed in these terms, the infrastructure for a neighborhood-based total population system has arguably been under development for decades—since the 1977 passage of the Community Reinvestment Act. The CRA aimed to democratize the availability of lending capital, initially for housing and small businesses, in low-income and racially segregated neighborhoods. Since its passage, it has evolved considerably into an important tool that underpins the work of people like David Erickson at the Federal Reserve and Douglas Jutte with the Build Healthy Places Network. The community development industry works directly with community groups and organizations to define capital requirements and design complex projects with layered financing from multiple sources (e.g., a building with a job training service, grocery store, and clinic within it). Community development pioneers have actively worked to build higher quality affordable housing that improves urban environments and the health of occupants (e.g., Jonathan Rose Companies). However, this sort of work has historically been disconnected from sources of healthcare financing. As healthcare systems shift to alternative payment models, leading community development institutions are exploring how their decades of experience in devising complex financial transactions can improve the value-proposition of neighborhood services and shift healthcare funds to the most effective among them.

As these financial pathways are being developed, the 100M Campaign is working to build the interpersonal, interorganizational relationships that will orchestrate their use. Their diverse membership is beginning to identify issues like homelessness that inherently cross sectors—housing, healthcare, public health, employment readiness, and criminal justice—all of which function differently, but will grow in capacity when they behave cooperatively. With the development of collateral pathways for "cheap talk" between traditionally gridlocked or noncommunicating actors—the chief aim of the 100M Community Health Improvement Academy and its collaborative means of achieving "rough consensus"—unprecedented system architectures will undoubtedly emerge to take advantage of new connectivity and relationships. It could take decades for a coherent total population health system to emerge from these promising components, but meanwhile the (not so) simple act of defining these components will enable the voices and actions of its citizen-members to take on a central role in animating the process.

So what happens when you step out of the abstract language of systems and into the neighborhood itself? How does one take these system tenets and turn them into a "feasible concept and an executable program"?

Enter Harlem.

12

Imagining the Future Out Loud

Once we open the door to the democratic implications of caregiving as moral and political practices, so much of the rest of our world from leadership to governance and from domestic to foreign affairs becomes a matter not just of markets, regulations, and security concerns, but of how we can enact care as humankind's shared project.
—Arthur Kleinman, "Caregiving as Moral Experience"

ARCHITECTING BETTER HEALTH IN HARLEM

The Harlem summer of 2015 promised to be just as warm as the summer of 2011, when I had started my medical internship. It had been four years since I first met Ray, and the neighborhood where he had grown up already felt different from the one he had left when he died.

In January 2015, HHS secretary Sylvia Burwell announced that Medicare reimbursements would be shifting from volume (fee-for-service) to value (alternative payment models) in gradual increments with a goal of 50 percent of Medicare dollars in value-based payment models by 2018. To facilitate a fundamental shift in strategy for the healthcare sector, HHS endeavored to provide sufficient guidance for healthcare organizations to determine their positioning as the landscape changes. She further stated that 90 percent of Medicare dollars would be linked to either quality or value by the same year.[1] Like ports extending conveyer belts into the sea to ease the journey of incoming ships, healthcare systems across the nation are entering the neighborhood where their patients live.

If Ray were alive today, he and his family would be encountering health systems like HHC and Mount Sinai Health System amidst paroxysms of change: both are actively working to improve accountability and quality in preparation for the shifts ahead. One such initiative, called Geriatric Emergency Department Innovations in Care through Workforce, Informatics, and Structural Enhancements (GEDI WISE),[2] has included City Health Works in its process design. An elderly diabetic discharged from Mount Sinai in 2015 is immediately matched up with a community health worker from City Health Works. This CHW not only ensures that he is taking his insulin dosage correctly, but also helps him understand how this medication relates to his diet and helps him anchor the management of his condition to more resonant life goals.

For New York healthcare systems like Mount Sinai, there is no turning back. On May 11, 2015, the New York State Department of Health informed the Mount Sinai Health System that it would be responsible for using $389 million of Delivery System Reform Incentive Payment (DSRIP) financing to redesign care for low-income New Yorkers. As we learned in chapter 8, DSRIP came into existence through a federal waiver that would change the way New York State administers Medicaid. This sum would have to be shared among a range of social services and neighborhood-level organizations, together comprising a Performing Provider System (PPS). The DSRIP financing would be available for five years (2015–20), with a growing emphasis on performance- and value-based outcomes. In theory, the financing would be administered through shared, coordinated, and connected infrastructure that integrated the work of more than 200 partners. Without a set of clear rules, and with little evidence to guide what combinations of overlapping processes might yield improved health outcomes or lower cost, individual PPSs, which comprise hundreds of organizations that overlap with their regional competitors, have to collectively find their way to a neighborhood-based health system that delivers results for low-income New Yorkers. The lead healthcare system in each PPS will not succeed without making sense of, and conducing cooperation across, the intra-organizational network. Hence the necessity for a new kind of hybrid workforce—part healthcare, part human services, locally hired and professionally trained—to make high-quality connections with neighbors at risk of poor health. The Greater New York Hospital Association (GNYHA) projects that the growth of population health models like New York State's DSRIP and Cambridge Health Alliance's PCMH will lead to substantial growth in new neighborhood-based health workforces, including a nearly exponential increase in the number of community health workers and more than doubling the number of health coaches.[3]

Labor organizations that have a significant presence in New York have already taken notice. For example, SEIU has rapidly forged links with 25 different PPSs to ensure that they would play a significant role in new, neighborhood-based workforce training.[4] Unlike during the historic clash decades ago (see chapter 2), they now have many points of connection and avenues for "cheap talk," which allow them to negotiate substantive differences with a network of organizational and political intermediaries. At the same time, New York City's Department of Health and Mental Hygiene (NYC-DOHMH) has begun ramping up its own community health worker initiative as part of its new Center for Health Equity, with a focus on East Harlem.

It was in this dynamic context that Rob Carmona, who organized the application to the 100M Campaign on behalf of the Harlem Hub, came to learn about DSRIP. His organization, Strive International, was connected to both SEIU and Mount Sinai as a catalyst for developing career pipelines into healthcare; Carmona had also caught wind of the NYCDOHMH's efforts. As healthcare systems planned for a significant move toward neighborhood-based care, buzz was spreading about new jobs, relationships, and responsibilities. Everyone had an angle to work.

The Harlem organizations that had applied to join the 100M Campaign as pacesetters persisted even when they were not selected for the SCALE initiative. They sought a scaffold to learn how to be a health organization, and the skills to position themselves with the foresight to navigate a rapidly shifting population health landscape. A Harlem-based organization like Strive, which does not see itself as a healthcare organization per se, needs guidance on where and how to fit into a total population health system whose parameters for outcomes, value, performance, and accountability have yet to be established. Strive's leaders know the needs and motivations of its members, both as people seeking careers in health and as neighbors serving as caregivers for their families. If the Mount Sinai Health System can integrate both perspectives—the professional perspective and the citizen-member perspective—into its PPS architecture, it will transform a clunky state-level initiative into a powerful periscope for life in the neighborhood.

Thanks in part to the efforts of people like Carmona, neighborhood intermediaries are emerging in Harlem. Intermediaries like Strive International serve as local routers that connect to multiple services, ranging from clinical care to employment opportunities and housing services. At the level of individuals, intermediaries like City Health Works's health coaches or Health Leads's volunteers help their clients match local assets to their needs. However, there are a lot of unknowns about how to efficiently coordinate their activities and manage their accountability to the people they serve. That said, their ability to cross the budget and information walls that thwart traditional healthcare systems and social services is considerable. As they mature and succeed in an evolving set of roles, they can add significant leadership and organizational skills to achieve common goals.[5]

The emergence of a new class of neighborhood intermediaries comes at a pivotal moment politically as well. The historic Harlem neighborhoods, including Washington Heights and parts of the Bronx, were organizing themselves in advance of a congressional race—the first open congressional race in 40 years—that presaged a colossal shakeup of political alliances, economic relationships, and social structure of the district. With Congressman Rangel stepping aside after his near loss in 2012, this race marked the end of a political era that stretched back two generations, to Ray's life as a young veteran.

According to an unpublished analysis done by BlueLabs, the data-oriented political firm that helped chart the path to President Barack Obama's presidential victories, the successful candidate—among some dozen contenders—had to reach a voting base that is pluralistic on multiple dimensions of racial, socioeconomic, and demographic composition. This requires the co-development of an issue- and coalition-based political platform, as compared to a historic reliance on sufficient voting turnout from a loyal base and a static network of allies honed over decades. The convergence of regional healthcare reform and the change in the social and political structure of Harlem is not just an important coincidence. The scaffold-building, coordinating work to be done by the Mount Sinai Health System PPS, Harlem neighborhood intermediaries, and the political candidates vying to represent the 13th District in Congress is sure to overlap, offering Harlem's citizen-members a rare opportunity to bring the professional, economic, and political imperatives of the neighborhood health system into alignment. Will anyone recognize the opportunities when they appear?

AMPLIFYING HARLEM'S VOICE

On June 18, 2015, I attended a community meeting at Taino Towers in East Harlem, where Strive happens to be located. The host of the meeting, Maria

Cruz, opened the evening with an emphatic sentiment in Spanish: *"Basta Ya!"* (Enough is enough). She asked her community to stop waiting for solutions to daily challenges from elected politicians and, instead, to clearly identify them and partner with those who have presented ways forward. The speakers, ranging from the police precinct chief, the district leader (one of over two dozen block-level leaders in the congressional district), and Clyde Williams, spoke about work they had underway to address local concerns. Williams introduced a petition to move forward legislation currently languishing in the state capitol in Albany to limit the density of drug abuse treatment and recovery facilities in a neighborhood.

Health and healthcare was a common theme throughout, including from the vantage point of the precinct chief, who wondered aloud if there could be more mental health support and ways to improve safety without arresting people. In the lively town hall–style exchange, the audience shared their proposed solutions and wanted to know whom they could hold accountable for meeting them. Some simply stated what they were doing and wanted to make sure that others knew about the opportunities they were creating. The exchange evoked the concept of a "culture of health" that RWJF had sought to foster across the nation, where the exchange of stories and experience created a shared meaning for the problems that the neighborhood had to face together.

I was invited to the Taino Towers event to share a project I was working on with a colleague, Stella Safo. We were prototyping an initiative called Harlem First, inspired by the work ISAIAH had done in Minnesota and grounded in the perspectives shared in *When People Come First*.[6] We had begun to do 1:1 sessions with members of the neighborhood to elicit their concerns and activate their involvement in the growing Harlem Hub. Williams, who was gathering signatures to move legislation that would reduce the density of the nearby methadone clinics, had put me in touch with Cruz so that we could present what we had learned and build further interest. To explain the purpose of Harlem First, I shared one powerful fact that continues to motivate me: a baby born in East Harlem today will live nearly a decade less than a baby born in neighborhoods closer to downtown Manhattan.[7] As if to drive this point home, a baby in the audience let loose a shrill cry. After the event, audience members showed overwhelming interest in both participating in 1:1s and learning how to do them in their blocks, places of worship, or organizations.

During the Harlem First 1:1s, Safo and I were listening keenly for how our neighbors framed challenges to their health and livelihood, as well as the promising ways forward that they were motivated to act upon. As we met community organizers who could train many others in the 1:1 format, we shifted our attention to how this information could be amplified and used by candidates for district leader to identify block-level challenges their constituents faced. We had three goals: (1) direct our neighbors to actions that would engage and leverage ongoing healthcare, public health, and neighborhood development initiatives that aligned with their goals; (2) create an evolving health and social policy platform to shape the views of neighborhood intermediaries and political candidates based upon Robert Putnam's premise that "the latent public support for addressing the underlying issue will become an irresistible 'market' for ambitious political candidates"[8]; and (3) map the conversation and supporting meta-data as it unfolded in an accessible way. In (1), my neighbors can affirmatively engage programs and services that fit their goals, while in (2), they have the means to drive wholesale reconsideration of their design through a democratic process. As we co-design (3) in ways that are meaningful to my neighbors, we discover ways to institutionalize progress and recognize opportunities. In all cases, communities with shared interests can form channels for dialogue and action, creating social capital in the process, which may itself be essential to better health. If Harlem First is the rudimentary path toward a collective sense for what health improvement means at the neighborhood level, then the practices like 1:1s, MI, and town halls are the vehicles for defining a shared purpose.

Although Safo and I continue to search for social and civic technology that fits our aims to develop a total population–level form of networking, we began with primitive tools: face-to-face interactions, documented using pen and paper. We then shared our goals with local social entrepreneurs and designers, who are eager to develop connective tools and methods for use on both the PPS systemwide level and the level of individual neighbors who make up the system. Our challenge, among others, will be scaling the process in ways that maintain the deeply personal nature of engagement, so that amplifying the voice and mapping the perspectives of any population whose health is to be managed becomes a healthcare system's point of entry to the neighborhoods it serves. Fortunately, there are healthcare leaders in and around Harlem who are increasingly adept at working with neighborhood organizations, who are being forged together by the context that DSRIP has created.

Within the Mount Sinai PPS, the weight of responsibility to interact with these dense networks within the neighborhood channel sits on the shoulders of Arthur Gianelli. Gianelli had had a decade of experience in public service at the county level, which earned him the moniker "budget wizard" by the *New York Times*,[9] before successfully leading a healthcare system with a substantial underserved population to expand its access. As the leader of the Mount Sinai PPS, Gianelli recognizes his role as a steward of public resources that have been thrust into a governance structure that is polycentric by definition, yet continues to search for the logic that will enable it to act collectively for population health. For Harlem to have a neighborhood-based health system that truly works for its diverse population, multiple PPSs will need to find common ways to interact with their partners, perhaps through connective systems like PCCI, which could simultaneously upgrade the data capabilities of many social sector organizations. There is a strong case for why state IT requirements should focus on this goal, perhaps in combination with pooled financing from CDFIs to create a HITECH act for New York City's social sector. This upgrade would accelerate the ability of all PPS partners to focus on their collective quality, identify empirical gaps in accountability, and shift investment to partners that can continuously improve their performance.

Even as the gap between the healthcare system and the neighborhood closes, the distance between their respective cultures and technologies is magnified. For an initiative like Harlem First to endure, it must be a purposeful instrument for its participants. Safo and I see it in its current incarnation as cohering a shared understanding of how my neighbors perceive their health in the context of their lives, locating the issues they see as interconnected with it, and finding ways to turn my neighbors' voices into action. These goals will undoubtedly evolve—or even be replaced—as experience dictates. More importantly, Harlem First must foster continuous discourse with systems that bear upon it, including but not limited to healthcare. In turn, whoever chooses to listen—the people who are running for elected office, neighborhood-based organizations in the PPS, community developers, and public health stewards—will have not only the statistics, descriptions, and data about important issues but the names and stories of local champions who are motivated to co-create solutions. Feedback across healthcare's neighborhood transoms will undoubtedly be rudimentary at first, but healthcare professionals have an enduring responsibility to keep the population they serve informed of the shifting landscape of health around them.

It is inevitable, and even essential, that many issues that emerge through the Harlem First initiative will have no cognate solution within healthcare systems as we know them, or will ever know them in the future. These issues may have primary implications for educational systems, in the case of adult literacy, or for deeper social discourse, in the case of racial inequity, or for more scalable systems to address depression and anxiety, which overwhelm our healthcare system capacity across the nation. This space between what formal healthcare systems offer and what people need to live healthier lives is the space that the 100M Campaign inhabits, spreading outward through its COIN and hub structures, which in turn enable channels of different shapes and sizes to exist so long as they are needed and supported by people who recognize their importance. It is the same space inhabited by the 100M application to form the Harlem Hub, which formed spontaneously and served as a virtual place for initiatives and organizations that logically *should* connect, but had not as yet. Given an arena for the "cheap talk" that makes meaningful relationships possible, neighborhood organizations and intermediaries have a platform to coordinate and engage with each other in unprecedented alliances.

At the same time, an NYC regional hub has been created, co-led by Rosanne Haggerty of Community Solutions. She, too, was present at the Baltimore 100 Million Healthier Lives Summit, and with the NYC Hub she brings together organizations that are working on homelessness, ranging from real estate experts to job training programs. The NYC and Harlem Hub do not connect in a hierarchal way, nor does the veterans health or child health hub, but they do have connections between them, and to hubs across the nation that can contribute unique expertise and ideas to address challenges articulated on all scales, from Medicare overhaul to DSRIP to Harlem First. There is no guarantee that a COIN of any size will persist, but their active formation increases the possibility of discovering unmet needs with resources at hand.

THE VALUE OF DESIGNING IN THE NEIGHBORHOOD

Imagine a perfect world in which a high-performing healthcare system and a healthier life in the neighborhood are synonymous, in which a total population health system, powered by polycentric governance, engages all of its citizen-members in achieving optimal health outcomes. How are such outcomes to be measured? How do we value the processes that produced them? In 1996, Santa Fe Institute economist W. Brian Arthur published a seminal article in *Harvard Business Review* called "Increasing Returns and the New World of Business," where he contrasted a traditional world of planning, hierarchy, and control with a new one of observation, positioning, and flattened organizations.[10] In the former, he argued, there are diminishing returns, where finite resources are consumed in accordance with available inputs; at some point, a hospital cannot operate without a certain level of payment for their services. In this context, it is crucial to focus on efficiency and optimization, which bear heavily upon the denominator—money—of how people think about value in healthcare. However, in the latter—a world governed by observation, positioning, and flattened organizations—there are new opportunities to combine skills, assets, and perspectives, opening up possibilities for unexpected abundance and strength as new structures and logics emerge to address a challenge at hand.

These emergent paradigms will either endure as new organizational forms or dissipate as goals are achieved. In this context, resources are in constant supply from an ever-changing array of sources, and collective solutions that emerge add value to all. If any neighborhood organizations (public or private) acted as part of a high-quality public health system they would systematically contribute to the numerator—better health outcomes. However, we focus far more on demanding incremental healthcare system efficiencies that change the denominator of the value equation (dollars spent) than on seeing the neighborhood as a channel that can dramatically increase the numerator (health improvement). As Arthur puts it, the former is a world of diminishing returns as resources are consumed; the latter leads to increasing returns as its network strengthens, its agile structure rapidly adapting to local needs.

How, then, can healthcare systems that are driven by the demands of quarterly financial performance contribute to, rather than resist, health improvement—driven value? Perhaps not coincidentally, Arthur's article was published on the heels of another seminal *Harvard Business Review* piece by Columbia Business School organizational theorist Rita Gunther McGrath, who introduced the concept of discovery-driven planning in 1995 (reintroduced as "discovery-driven growth" in 2009).[11] In discovery-driven planning, decisions must change as new information is revealed. Nowhere is this concept more useful than in the profound uncertainty of how DSRIP will unfold in the context of a new generation of population health business models. Conventional, quarter-by-quarter financial planning is likely to lead to significant under-investments in new partnerships, positions, and processes that are crucial to the sustainability of healthcare systems.

Addressing the challenge of investing in the future when there is no formula for organizing such investments, McGrath argues that "enhancement launches," like a movement from volume to value by healthcare systems, and "platform launches," such as engaging the DSRIP initiative to build a partnership structure, are necessary for incremental reinvention and reinvestment. Gathering insights from business leaders who have engaged in such practices, she found that opportunity arises from three different types of options. The first, "scouting options," occurs where a healthcare system looks for opportunities to use its existing capabilities in new ways as its context changes (e.g., improving quality of neighborhood partners in a PPS, which leads to new collective capabilities). A second type, "positioning options," occurs where a healthcare system finds promising contexts to build new capabilities (e.g., investing in civic and social technologies to improve engagement with population health services). The third type could be characterized as effort-limited "stepping stones," which are incremental opportunities to change the underlying fundamentals of healthcare (e.g., investing in Harlem First as a social feedback loop for healthcare system design).

As McGrath says, it is possible to build a strategy by imagining a future state and working backward. Accordingly, a healthier future doesn't start with how to pay for it. What comes first is the neighborhood developing a shared view of what a healthier life could be. Only then can communities begin to figure out how to get the most from every dollar spent to improve health. What's important is imagining it out loud.[12]

The will to develop new organizational behaviors that are pro-social and pro-health requires ideas and vision. However, money matters and healthcare's prevailing economic logic shape organizational behavior. More needs to be learned, by doing, to translate Arthur's logic of increasing returns to population health. The most important step forward requires liberalizing the type of entities that are eligible for healthcare financing in order to reflect the diversity of organizations that can contribute to a greater numerator in the value equation. This process must be carefully structured and monitored, lest the avenues of fraud and abuse, which are already rampant among traditional healthcare entities, spread into new forms. More importantly, the rigid methods for measuring and attributing health improvement to pills and procedures should evolve to identify and improve upon networks of coordinated neighborhood activity, rather than silver-bullet interventions alone. Some of the most promising work is in the arenas of childhood health and development, where the concept of *scaffolds* is a powerful way to integrate multiple methods, insights, and disciplines, and in heart health, where positive attributes of cardiovascular well-being and preventive health sit on a testable continuum with chronic conditions and acute illness.[13] Both of these areas reflect avenues where experts can begin to grapple with the complexity of what it means to grow up and stay healthy in a dynamic neighborhood.

There are other avenues forward, if we as a nation are bold enough to take them. What if we sought to tally the total healthcare system spending in every neighborhood and the health outcomes it yielded? Such a sum would represent the total value proposition for the current way that healthcare and public health and neighborhood organizations are organized. We should encourage a learning network of places across America (the observation component of Arthur's value system of increasing returns) to take on the risk of developing new modes of mutual accountability (planning), particularly if they have a track record of inclusivity and collaboration (as a flat organization with many types of assets).

For this to work, federal and state rules that govern public healthcare and social sector financing would have to be modified for a self-identified group of places that could participate in a SCALE-like learning network. Places like Hennepin County, Minnesota, where Hennepin Health has forged together multiple organizational types, are already scouting out the expertise and experience to lead the way. Of the 200,000 neighborhoods across the country, only a fraction would have the right mix of experience, know-how, and cohesiveness to consider this approach. As it should be: these pioneer neighborhoods would generate formative learning to inform a more refined and technically rigorous process that could spread if successful. These efforts should yield a new class of social and civic technologies that lead to better health and a healthier neighborhood, where Arthur defines technologies as the means for fulfilling a human purpose, composed of an assemblage of interrelated components and a collection of engineering practices available to a culture.[14] Today, artificial barriers between health-care financing and the rest of our economy stymie our ability to truly engage our neighbors in a search for high-value healthcare that is in sync with a healthier neighborhood. If my neighbors were welcomed as co-architects, I have no doubt that their perspectives would radically reshape its design to a neighborhood-based health system that could connect more intimately with our needs as human beings.

In moving forward, we must share in the purposes of the neighborhood, which reside in its many voices, improve upon the assemblages that produc-tively channel them, and create shared practices to tinker with the architec-ture of healthcare systems that are shared by experts and neighbors alike.

DESIGNING FROM WITHIN A HEALTHCARE SYSTEM

Months before my residency came to a close on June 30, 2015, I had resolved to take a more active role in my neighborhood when it ended. The people and organizations I had encountered across the country, and within my neighborhood, led me to believe that far from being an era of disillusion-ment for my profession, it was a time of unprecedented opportunity to shift our internal gaze outward. In practical terms, that meant recommitting to learning and discovering how to improve the life of people in the neigh-borhoods we serve, with full application of our economic heft, political influence, and analytic capabilities.

The opportunity to be involved in this transformation was forthcoming: I committed to joining the Mount Sinai Health System as Vice Chairman of Medicine for Population Health and leading its Arnhold Institute, which will focus on global population health. Around the same time, the Mount Sinai Health System released a series of full-page *New York Times* adver-tisements, including one boldly declaring, "If our hospital beds are filled, it means we've failed." In this committed environment, I began working with the system's leadership to redesign how financial, technological, workforce, and clinical processes contribute to the total population health of the neigh-borhoods we serve. Fortunately, we join a growing number of healthcare systems nationwide that are on the same journey.

As a member of an academic medical center, part of my role is to search for and bring to light important questions in partnership with talented and dedicated colleagues. As I continue work as a primary care doctor, I am certain these questions will necessarily include the very nature of how we are organized in relation to the goals of my neighbors. For healthcare systems to appreciate the latter, they must build deeply integrated partnerships with the former. More importantly, the empathy that we speak of as being important at the level of individuals must become systemic. Together, we must commit to improve the design, performance, and architecture of a total population health system—a system that makes visible the constraints in our daily lives and co-creates the conditions that enable all of us to flourish.

Notes

Preface

Epigraph. Rudolph Virchow, *Standpoint in Scientific Medicine*, 1848

1. John C. Burnham, "American Medicine's Golden Age: What Happened to It?" *Science* 215, no. 4539 (1982): 1474–79, DOI:10.1126/science.7038876.

2. Sandeep Jauhar, "Why Doctors Are Sick of Their Profession," *Wall Street Journal*, August 29, 2014, http://online.wsj.com/articles/the-u-s-s-ailing-medical-system-a -doctors-perspective-1409325361.

3. J. R. Ashton (with acknowledgements to Siân Anis), "Virchow Misquoted, Part-Quoted, and the Real McCoy," *Journal of Epidemiology and Community Health* 60, no. 8 (2006): 671. http://www.ncbi.nlm.nih.gov/pmc/articles/PMC2588080.

4. Theodore M. Brown and Elizabeth Fee, "Rudolf Carl Virchow," *American Journal of Public Health* 96, no. 12 (1996): 2104–5, DOI: 10.2105/AJPH.2005.078436.

5. Ibid., p. 2104.

6. Russ Roberts, *Jeffrey Sachs on the Millennium Villages Project*. Web Interview. *EconTalk*, March 17, 2014.

7. Michael Bliss, *William Osler: A Life in Medicine* (Oxford University Press, 2007).

Introduction

Epigraph. Committee on Quality of Health Care in America, Institute of Medicine, *Crossing the Quality Chasm: A New Health System for the 21st Century* (National Academies Press, 2001).

1. Martin Gaynor, Kate Ho, and Robert Town, "The Industrial Organization of Health Care Markets," National Bureau of Economic Research Working Paper No. 19800 (2014), DOI: 10.3386/w19800.

2. Moses Hamilton III, D. H. Matheson, E. R. Dorsey, B. P. George, D. Sadoff, and S. Yoshimura, "The Anatomy of Health Care in the United States," *JAMA* 310, no. 18 (2013): 1947–64, DOI:10.1001/jama.2013.281425.

3. Horst W. J. Rittel and Melvin M. Webber, "Dilemmas in a General Theory of Planning," *Policy Sciences* 4 (1973): 155–69, http://www.uctc.net/mwebber/Rittel +Webber+Dilemmas+General_Theory_of_Planning.pdf.

4. Amitabh Chandra, Jonathan Holmes, and Jonathan Skinner. "Is This Time Different? The Slowdown in Healthcare Spending," NBER Working Paper 19700 (2013).

5. Samantha Smith, "From the Very Start, Sharp Partisan Divisions over Obamacare," Pew Research Center, June 25, 2015.

6. http://www.pewresearch.org/fact-tank/2015/06/25/from-the-very-start-sharp -partisan-divisions-over-obamacare/.

7. Alfred Marshall, *Principles of Economics* (1890), https://www.marxists.org /reference/subject/economics/marshall/bk4ch10.htm.

8. G. Thomas Kingsley, Claudia J. Coulton, and Kathryn L. S. Pettit, *Strengthening Communities with Neighborhood Data* (Urban Institute, 2014), http://www.urban.org /sites/default/files/13805_urban-kingsley.pdf.

9. Gina Kolata, "Genes Take Charge, and Diets Fall by the Wayside," *New York Times*, May 8, 2007, http://www.nytimes.com/2007/05/08/health/08fat.html?pagewanted =all and _r=0.

10. "Zip Code as Important as Genetic Code in Childhood Obesity," Seattle Children's Hospital Research Foundation, April 10, 2012, http://www.seattlechildrens.org /press-releases/2012/zip-code-as-important-as-genetic-code-in-childhood-obesity/.

11. Diabetes Prevention Program Research Group, "Reduction in the Incidence of Type 2 Diabetes with Lifestyle Intervention or Metformin," *New England Journal of Medicine* 346 (2002): 393–403, DOI: 10.1056/NEJMoa012512.

12. Charles E. Rosenberg, "Inward Vision and Outward Glance: The Shaping of the American Hospital, 1880–1914," *Bulletin of the History of Medicine* 53, no. 3 (1979): 346–91. Rosenberg went on to write, "Such behavior is not comprehensible in purely material terms. The honor accorded to innovation, the satisfaction of intellectual competence in a world of pervasive mediocrity, for example, are meaningful compensations—if perhaps no more transcendent than dollars and cents (and possibly more self-deluding). One can hardly understand the evolution of the hospital without some understanding of the power of ideas, of the allure of innovation, of the promise of healing, of the amelioration of painful and incapacitating symptoms through an increasingly hospital-based technology."

13. M. Maier and E. Rechtin, *The Art of Systems Architecting*, 3rd ed. (CRC Press, 2009).

14. Roger Cohen, "From Death into Life," *New York Times*, April 7, 2014.

Chapter 1. Out of Many, One

Epigraph. Langston Hughes, "Night Funeral in Harlem" in *The Collected Poems of Langston Hughes* (Alfred A. Knopf, 1994).

1. HealthData.gov, *http://www.healthdata.gov/blog/building-healthy-community -technology-and-community-members*—launched in 2012, with very limited distribution as part of the Primary Care Information Project.

2. Rishi Manchanda's *The Upstream Doctors* in "Investigating the root causes of the global health crisis: Paul Farmer on the TED Book 'The Upstream Doctors,'" TED Blog, http://blog.ted.com/investigating-the-root-causes-of-the-global-health-crisis-paul -farmer-on-the-upstream-doctors.

3. "The Sesquicentennial, 1852–2002," Mount Sinai Hospital, p. 13, http://library .mssm.edu/services/archives/pdf/150_booklet.pdf.

4. Ibid.

5. Sam Grobart, "Dr. Freeman: War on Poverty," *New York Magazine*, 1999, http:// nymag.com/nymetro/health/bestdoctors/features/590/.

6. Harold P. Freeman, M.D., "Cancer in the Economically Disadvantaged," *Cancer* 64 (July 1989): 324–34, published online in 2006, http://onlinelibrary.wiley.com/doi

/10.1002/1097-0142%2819890701%2964:1%2B%3C324::AID-CNCR2820641334%3E3.0.CO;2-B/full.

7. Michael Sterne, "In Last Decade, Leaders Say Harlem's Dreams Have Died," *New York Times*, March 1, 1978, http://vergara.nyhistory.org/wp-content/uploads/2012/05/Harlems-Dreams-Have-Died-NYTimes-1978-2.pdf.

8. Grobart, "Dr. Freeman."

9. Colin McCord, M.D., and Harold P. Freeman, M.D., "Excess Mortality in Harlem," *New England Journal of Medicine* 322, no. 3 (1990): 173–77, http://www.nejm.org/doi/pdf/10.1056/NEJM199001183220306.

10. Harold P. Freeman, M.D., and Rian L. Rodriguez, M.P.H., "History and Principles of Patient Navigation," *Cancer* 117 (August 2011): 3537–40.

11. Ibid.

12. Robert B. Vargas, M.D., M.P.H., Gery W. Ryan, Ph.D., Catherine A. Jackson, Ph.D., Rian Rodriguez, M.P.H., and Harold P. Freeman, M.D., "Characteristics of the Original Patient Navigation Programs to Reduce Disparities in the Diagnosis and Treatment of Breast Cancer," *Cancer* 113 (July 2008): 426–33, http://onlinelibrary.wiley.com/doi/10.1002/cncr.23547/epdf.

13. Prediabetes is not considered to be a clinical state, but it does refer to a set of risk factors that has a high probability of leading to diabetes, including obesity. The CDC has provided guidance in "Prediabetes: Am I at Risk?" Centers for Disease Control and Prevention, http://www.cdc.gov/diabetes/prevention/prediabetes.htm, accessed 2/16/2013.

14. See "Obesity in East and Central Harlem: A Look across Generations," New York City Department of Health and Hygiene, http://www.nyc.gov/html/doh/downloads/pdf/dpho/dpho-harlem-obesity.pdf.

15. Punam Parikh, M.P.H., Ellen P. Simon, D.S.W., Kezhen Fei, M.S., Helen Looker, M.D., Crispin Goytia, B.S., and Carol R. Horowitz, M.D., M.P.H., "Results of a Pilot Diabetes Prevention Intervention in East Harlem, New York City: Project HEED," *American Journal of Public Health* 100 (2010): S232–39, DOI: 10.2105/AJPH.2009.170910.

16. Jessica Y. Breland, M.S., Lisa M. McAndrew, Ph.D., Rachel L. Gross, B.A., Howard Leventhal, Ph.D., and Carol R. Horowitz, M.D., "Challenges to Healthy Eating for People with Diabetes in a Low-Income, Minority Neighborhood," *Diabetes Care* (2013), DOI: 10.2337/dc12-1632.

17. Rebecca Onie, "What If Our Healthcare System Kept Us Healthy? TED Talk, June 2012, https://www.ted.com/talks/rebecca_onie_what_if_our_healthcare_system_kept_us_healthy?language=en.

18. This widely cited quote was from a speech given in 1965. See http://www.cse.umd.edu/blog/-from-diagnosis-to-social-diagnosis-a-social-scientists-guide-to-diagnosing-environmental-health-problems.

19. Susan Sontag, *Illness as Metaphor and Aids and Its Metaphors* (Doubleday, 1990).

20. Herbert Muschamp, "Architecture as an Antidote," *New York Times*, September

24, 1992, http://www.nytimes.com/1992/09/24/nyregion/architecture-as-an-antidote
.html.

21. Paul Bergl, M.D., "Medical Interns—Not at the Bedside, but Not to Be Blamed,"
NEJM Journal Watch, September 16, 2013, http://blogs.jwatch.org/general-medicine
/index.php/2013/09/medical-interns-not-at-the-bedside/.

22. Michel Foucault, "Docile Bodies," and "The Means of Correct Training" in *The
Foucault Reader*, ed. Paul Rabinow (Pantheon, 1984), p. 23.

23. Steven A. Schroeder. "We Can Do Better—Improving the Health of the American People," *New England Journal of Medicine* 357, no. 12 (2007): 1221–28.

24. Katherine Baicker, Ph.D., Sarah L. Taubman, Sc.D., Heidi L. Allen, Ph.D., Mira
Bernstein, Ph.D., Jonathan H. Gruber, Ph.D., Joseph P. Newhouse, Ph.D., Eric C.
Schneider, M.D., Bill J. Wright, Ph.D., Alan M. Zaslavsky, Ph.D., and Amy N. Finkel-
stein, Ph.D. for the Oregon Health Study Group, "The Oregon Experiment—Effects of
Medicaid on Clinical Outcomes," *New England Journal of Medicine* 368, no.18 (2013):
1713–22, DOI: 10.1056/NEJMsa1212321; Amy Finkelstein, Sarah Taubman, Bill Wright,
Mira Bernstein, Jonathan Gruber, Joseph P. Newhouse, Heidi Allen, Katherine Baicker,
and the Oregon Health Study Group, "The Oregon Health Insurance Experiment:
Evidence from the First Year," *Quarterly Journal of Economics* 127, no. 3 (2012):
1057–1106, DOI:10.1093/qje/qjs020.

25. Raymond Fisman, "Straining Emergency Rooms by Expanding Health Insurance," *Science* 343, no. 6168 (2014): 252–53, DOI: 10.1126/science.1249341.

26. Joshua J. Fenton, M.D., M.P.H., Anthony F. Jerant, M.D., Klea D. Bertakis, M.D.,
M.P.H., Peter Franks, M.D., "The Cost of Satisfaction: A National Study of Patient
Satisfaction, Health Care Utilization, Expenditures, and Mortality," *JAMA Internal
Medicine* 172, no. 5 (2012): 405–11, DOI:10.1001/archinternmed.2011.1662.

Chapter 2. Heads in Beds

Epigraph. David Stark, *The Sense of Dissonance: Accounts of Worth in Economic Life*
(Princeton University Press, 2011).

1. Ellen Gustafson. *We the Eaters: If We Change Dinner, We Can Change the World*
(Rodale Press, 2014).

2. Healthy People.gov, Health and Human Services, http://www.healthypeople.gov/.

3. Prabhjot Singh and Jeffrey D. Sachs, "1 Million Community Health Workers
in Sub-Saharan Africa by 2015," *Lancet* 382, no. 9889 (2013): 363–65, DOI: http://
dx.doi.org/10.1016/S0140-6736(12)62002-9.

4. Prabhjot Singh, M.D., Ph.D., and Dave A. Chokshi, M.D., "Community Health
Workers—A Local Solution to a Global Problem," *New England Journal of Medicine*
369 (2013): 894–96, DOI: 10.1056/NEJMp1305636.

5. At the time of his death, Ray was "dual-eligible" for both Medicaid and Medicare.

6. Diana Rodin, M.P.H., and Jack Meyer, Ph.D., "Health Care Costs and Spending
in New York State, New York State Health Foundation, February 2014, http://nyshealth
foundation.org/uploads/resources/health-care-costs-in-NYS-chart-book.pdf.

7. "A Plan to Transform the Empire State's Medicaid Program: Better Care, Better Health, Lower Costs," New York State Department of Health, https://www.health.ny .gov/health_care/medicaid/redesign/docs/mrtfinalreport.pdf.

8. Adam Reich, *Selling Our Souls: The Commodification of Hospital Care in the United States* (Princeton University Press, 2014), p. 21.

9. Donald M. Berwick, M.D., "Reshaping US Health Care from Competition and Confiscation to Cooperation and Mobilization," *JAMA* 312, no. 20 (2014): 2099–2100, DOI:10.1001/jama.2014.15727.

10. Karen E. Joynt, M.D., M.P.H., E. John Orav, Ph.D., and Ashish K. Jha, M.D., M.P.H., "Association between Hospital Conversions to For-Profit Status and Clinical and Economic Outcomes," *JAMA* 312, no.16 (2014): 1644–52, DOI:10.1001/jama.2014.13336.

11. "Variation in Standards and Guidance Limits Comparison of How Hospitals Meet Community Benefit Requirements," GAO, http://www.gao.gov/new.items /d08880.pdf.

12. Gary J. Young, J.D., Ph.D., Chia-Hung Chou, Ph.D., Jeffrey Alexander, Ph.D., Shoou-Yih Daniel Lee, Ph.D., and Eli Raver, "Provision of Community Benefits by Tax-Exempt U.S. Hospitals," *New England Journal of Medicine* 368 (2013): 1519–27, DOI: 10.1056/NEJMsa1210239 (this includes religious organizations); Sara Rosenbaum, Amber Rieke, and Maureen Byrnes, "Hospital Community Benefit Expenditures: Looking behind the Numbers," *Health Affairs Blog*, http://healthaffairs.org/blog/2013 /06/11/hospital-community-benefit-expenditures-looking-behind-the-numbers.

13. Dan Goldberg, "De Blasio's Surgeon," *Capital*, July 31, 2014, http://www .capitalnewyork.com/article/city-hall/2014/07/8549578/de-blasios-surgeon.

14. David Cutler, "The Health-Care Law's Success Story: Slowing Down Medical Costs," *Washington Post*, November 8, 2013, http://www.washingtonpost.com/opinions /the-health-care-laws-success-story-slowing-down-medical-costs/2013/11/08 /e08cc52a-47c1-11e3-b6f8-3782ff6cb769_story.html.

15. Medicare is a federally administered program and is more uniform than Medicaid, which is administered by the states with joint oversight over minimum eligibility that derives from federal standards. It varies considerably by state.

16. Tax breaks are larger than combined federal discretionary spending in the FY2015, but there is controversy surrounding how they should be counted, since their fiscal impact is much more difficult to trace. The federal budget in FY2015 is approximately 21 percent of the total US economy as defined by the gross domestic product, according to the nonpartisan Office of Management and Budget. From: "Federal Spending: Where Does Money Go," National Priorities Project, https://www .nationalpriorities.org/budget-basics/federal-budget-101/spending/.

17. Kenneth J. Arrow, "Uncertainty and the Welfare Economics of Medical Care," *American Economic Review* 53, no. 5 (1963): 941–73, quote on p. 943.

18. Farshad Fani Marvasti, M.D., M.P.H., and Randall S. Stafford, M.D., Ph.D., "From Sick Care to Health Care—Reengineering Prevention into the U.S. System," *New England Journal of Medicine* 367 (2012): 889–91, DOI: 10.1056/NEJMp1206230.

19. M. Hartman, A. B. Martin, J. Benson, A. Catlin, and the National Health Expenditure Accounts Team, "National Health Spending in 2011: Overall Growth Remains Low, but Some Payers and Services Show Signs of Acceleration," *Health Affairs* 32, no. 1 (2013): 87–99, DOI: 10.1377/hlthaff.2012.1206.

20. Martin Gaynor, Kate Ho, and Robert J. Town, "The Industrial Organization of Health Care Markets," National Bureau of Economic Research, Working Paper No. 19800 (2014), https://hcmg.wharton.upenn.edu/files/?whdmsaction=public:main.file&fileID=8079.

21. Arrow, "Uncertainty and the Welfare Economics of Medical Care," p. 947.

22. "2014 Milliman Medical Index," Milliman Research Report, http://www.milliman.com/uploadedFiles/insight/Periodicals/mmi/pdfs/2014-mmi.pdf.

23. David I. Auerbach and Arthur L. Kellermann, "A Decade of Health Care Cost Growth Has Wiped Out Real Income Gains for an Average US Family," *Health Affairs* 30, no. 9 (2011): 160–63, DOI: 10.1377/hlthaff.2011.0585.

24. Charles Roehrig. "U.S. Budget Implications: What if the Massachusetts Health Spending Goal Was Applied Nationally? Goal of GDP+0 Revisited." Blog. August 14, 2012. http://altarum.org/health-policy-blog/u-s-budget-implications-what-if-the-massachusetts-health-spending-goal-was-applied-nationally-goal.

25. "We are looking for the underlying reason that people are coming back to the hospital," said Maria Basso Lipani, program director for Mount Sinai's Preventable Admissions Care Team. "We really will do anything and everything." Quoted in Shannon Pettypiece, "Obamacare Keeps Patients at Home Slowing Hospital Use," *Bloomberg Business*, September 25, 2013, http://www.bloomberg.com/news/articles/2013-09-25/obamacare-keeps-patients-at-home-slowing-hospital-use.

26. Robert Kelley. "Where Can $700 Billion in Waste Be Cut Annually from the U.S. Healthcare System?" Thomson Reuters, October 2009, http://blr.healthleadersmedia.com/content/241965.pdf.

27. Michael E. Porter, Ph.D., "What Is Value in Health Care?" *New England Journal of Medicine* 363 (2010): 2477–81, quote on p. 2481, DOI: 10.1056/NEJMp1011024.

28. Ibid., p. 2477.

29. Kent J. Moore, Thomas A. Felger, M.D., Walter L. Larimore, M.D., and Terry L. Mills Jr., M.D., "What Every Physician Should Know about the RUC," *Family Practice Management* 15, no. 2 (2008): 36–39, http://www.aafp.org/fpm/2008/0200/p36.html#fpm20080200p36-b1.

30. Porter, "What Is Value in Health Care?" p. 2479.

31. "The Dartmouth Atlas of Healthcare," Dartmouth Institute for Health Policy and Clinical Practice, http://www.dartmouthatlas.org/data/region/.

32. "The 2010 Higley 1000," Higley 1000, http://higley1000.com/archives/638.

33. Jose A. DelReal, "Obamacare Consultant under Fire for 'Stupidity of the American Voter' comment," *Washington Post*, November 11, 2014, http://www.washingtonpost.com/blogs/post-politics/wp/2014/11/11/obamacare-consultant-under-fire-for-stupidity-of-the-american-voter-comment/.

34. The Health Indiana Plan required a complex waiver that significantly redesigns how Medicaid operates. More here: "Medicaid Expansion in Indiana," Henry J. Kaiser Family Foundation, February 3, 2015, http://kff.org/medicaid/fact-sheet/medicaid -expansion-in-indiana/.

35. Many did not know that their insurance product was inadequate until it became ineligible to participate in the exchange; the president got into trouble because of this.

36. "Facts and Figures," Mount Sinai, http://www.mountsinaihealth.org/about -the-health-system/facts-and-figures.

37. "Care about Your Care: Tips for Patients When They Leave the Hospital," Dartmouth Atlas of Health Care, http://www.dartmouthatlas.org/downloads/reports/Atlas _CAYC_092811.pdf.

38. Kenneth L. Davis, M.D., "Social Service Support: Better for Individuals and Health Care," Mount Sinai Hospital, http://www.mountsinai.org/static_files/MSMC /Files/NYT%20OpEds/MS_OpEd%20Ad_SocialService.pdf.

39. This is a complex debate: Ashish K. Jha, M.D., M.P.H., and Alan M. Zaslavsky, Ph.D., "Quality Reporting That Addresses Disparities in Health Care," *JAMA* 312, no. 3 (2014): 225–26, DOI:10.1001/jama.2014.7204.

40. Jordan Rau, "Medicare Fines 2,610 Hospitals in Third Round of Readmission Penalties," Kaiser Health News, October 2, 2014, http://kaiserhealthnews.org/news /medicare-readmissions-penalties-2015/.

41. Jianhui Hu, Meredith D. Gonsahn, and David R. Nerenz, "Socioeconomic Status and Readmissions: Evidence from an Urban Teaching Hospital," *Health Affairs* 33, no. 5 (2014): 778–85, DOI: 10.1377/hlthaff.2013.0816.

42. Robert Lenzner, "The Hospital of Tomorrow: Redefining Hospitals under the Affordable Care Act," *Forbes*, May 21, 2014, http://www.forbes.com/sites/robertlenzner /2014/05/21/the-hospital-of-tomorrow-redefining-hospitals-under-the-affordable -care-act/.

43. Julie Brill, "Competition in Health Care Markets" (keynote address at the Hal White Antitrust Conference, Washington D.C., June 9, 2014), http://www.ftc.gov /system/files/documents/public_statements/314861/140609halwhite.pdf.

Chapter 3. A Purposeful Neighborhood

Epigraph. W. Edwards Deming. *The New Economics for Industry, Government, Education* (MIT Press, 2000), p. 50.

1. Ibid.

2. Bengt Lindström and Monica Eriksson, "Salutogenesis," *Journal of Epidemiology and Community Health* 59, no. 6 (2005): 440–42, DOI:10.1136/jech.2005.034777.

3. Personal communication, Casabe House meeting, July 1, 2013.

4. Jonathan Gill, *Harlem: The Four Hundred Year History from Dutch Village to Capital of Black America* (Grove Press, 2012).

5. This understates the diversity of the neighborhood—Leonard Covello, author of

The Heart Is the Teacher (McGraw-Hill, 1958), estimated that there were 34 ethnicities speaking 27 languages in the neighborhood.

6. "National Affairs: Veto Vito?" *Time*, November 4, 1946, p. 25, http://content.time .com/time/magazine/article/0,9171,777181,00.html.

7. Christopher Bell, *East Harlem Remembered: Oral Histories of Community and Diversity* (McFarland, 2012), p. 96.

8. Ibid., p. 120.

9. Robert Caro later regretted having had to remove an entire chapter on Jacobs's activism against powerful urban planners in his authoritative account of the era in *The Power Broker: Robert Moses and the Fall of New York* (Knopf, 1974), according to Scott Porch in his article "'The Power Broker' Turns 40: How Robert Caro Wrote a Masterpiece," *Daily Beast*, September 16, 2014.

10. Hilary W. Hoynes, Diane Whitmore Schanzenbach, and Douglas Almond, "Long Run Impacts of Childhood Access to the Safety Net," National Bureau of Economic Research Working Paper No. 18535 (2012), http://www.nber.org/papers /w18535.

11. Roger Vaughan, "The Real Great Society," *Life* 63, no. 11 (1967): 80.

12. Union Settlement became one of the nation's first Head Start programs, in 1974, and was the site of a federal initiative for primary healthcare that still stands.

13. The powerful ethnographic work of anthropologist Philippe Bourgois, *In Search of Respect: Selling Crack in El Barrio*, 2nd ed. (Cambridge University Press, 2003) gives deeper insight into the psychology and dynamics of a neighborhood in decline.

14. David J. Erickson, *The Housing Policy Revolution: Networks and Neighborhoods* (Urban Institute Press, 2009), p. 254.

15. "Manhattan Community District 11," http://www.nyc.gov/html/dcp/pdf/lucds /mn11profile.pdf.

16. "Community Reinvestment Act (CRA)," *Board of Governors of the Federal Reserve System*, http://www.federalreserve.gov/communitydev/cra_about.htm—revised in 2005. "The CRA requires that each depository institution's record in helping meet the credit needs of its entire community be evaluated by the appropriate Federal financial supervisory agency periodically. Members of the public may submit comments on a bank's performance. Comments will be taken into consideration during the next CRA examination. A bank's CRA performance record is taken into account in considering an institution's application for deposit facilities."

17. Erickson, *The Housing Policy Revolution*, p. 18.

18. This has led to socially conscious developers and investors, such as the Jonathan Rose Companies and the Healthy Neighborhood Equity Fund, respectively. Despite the Federal Reserve's analysis, critics persist in tracing the CRA to the subprime mortgage crisis that contributed to the extended recession. See Paul Krugman, "Origins of the Crisis, Fake and Real," *New York Times*, May 21, 2011.

19. He was assassinated in Manhattan and died at Columbia-Presbyterian Hospital in 1965.

20. It also opened it up to questionable businesses that trade credits like stock options. See Erickson, *The Housing Policy Revolution*.

21. Melinda Henneberger, "Rangel's Voice: Stronger than Ever; Dean of Delegation Furious over Cuts," *New York Times*, May 16, 1995, http://www.nytimes.com/1995/05/16 /nyregion/rangel-s-voice-stronger-than-ever-dean-of-delegation-furious-over-cuts .html.

22. Elizabeth H. Bradley and Lauren A. Taylor, *The American Health Care Paradox: Why Spending More Is Getting Us Less* (Public Affairs, 2013). They use the OECD Social Expenditure Database, p. 109.

23. New York City Department of Health and Mental Hygiene, "Community Health Profiles, 2015: East Harlem" (http://www.nyc.gov/html/doh/downloads/pdf/data /2015chp-mn11.pdf), p. 6; "Central Harlem" (http://www.nyc.gov/html/doh/downloads /pdf/data/2015chp-mn10.pdf), p. 6. See these profiles for additional statistics on the neighborhoods.

24. Jacob S. Hacker, *The Divided Welfare State: The Battle over Public and Private Social Benefits in the United States* (Cambridge University Press, 2002), p. 16.

25. Jacob Funk Kirkegaard, "The True Levels of Government and Social Expenditures in Advanced Economies," *Peterson Institute for International Economics* Number PB 15-4 (2015), http://www.piie.com/publications/pb/pb15-4.pdf.

26. As quoted in John Freeman Gill, "Frederick Douglass Boulevard: Newly Revived," *New York Times*, December 31, 2013, http://mobile.nytimes.com/2014/01/05 /realestate/frederick-douglass-boulevard-newly-revived.html?referrer=and_r=0.

27. "Evidence Counts: Evaluating State Tax Incentives for Jobs and Growth," Pew Charitable Trusts, April 12, 2012, http://www.pewtrusts.org/~/media/assets/2012/04 /12/pew_evaluating_state_tax_incentives_report.pdf.

28. Tony Baragona, Alison Chiu, Kayla Loveman, Emma Marconi, Adam Poole, Susie Ranney, Sarah Ripple, and Myun Song, "East Harlem: Preserving the Working Man's Manhattan," http://www.arch.columbia.edu/files/gsapp/imceshared/East _Harlem_Studio_2011.pdf.

29. Literally—a study of amputation rates in California due to diabetes demonstrated that this terrible outcome clustered in low-income neighborhoods: Carl D. Stevens, David L. Schriger, Brian Raffetto, Anna C. Davis, David Zingmond, and Dylan H. Roby, "Geographic Clustering of Diabetic Lower-Extremity Amputations in Low-Income Regions of California," *Health Affairs* 33, no. 8 (2014): 1383–90, DOI: 10.1377/hlthaff.2014.0148.

30. Joseph Farrell and Matthew Rabin, "Cheap Talk," *Journal of Economic Perspectives* 10, no. 3 (1996): 103–18, http://www.jstor.org/stable/2138522?scq=1&#page_scan _tab_contents.

31. Elinor Ostrom, "Beyond Markets and States: Polycentric Governance of Complex Economic Systems," Nobel Prize Lecture, December 8, 2009, http://www.nobelprize .org/nobel_prizes/economic-sciences/laureates/2009/ostrom_lecture.pdf.

32. Elliott S. Fisher, M.D., M.P.H., and Janet Corrigan, Ph.D., "Accountable Health

Communities: Getting There from Here," *JAMA* 312, no. 20 (2014): 2093–94, DOI: 10.1001/jama.2014.13815.

33. Dan Buettner, *The Blue Zones: Lessons for Living Longer from the People Who've Lived the Longest* (National Geographic, 2010).

34. Mark W. Maier, *The Art of Systems Architecting*, 3rd ed. (CRC Press, 2009), p. 441.

Chapter 4. Contexts of Consequence

Epigraph. Deborah Solomon, "Health-Conscious: The Way We Live Now: 6-19-05: Questions for Richard Carmona," *New York Times Magazine*, June 19, 2005, http://www.nytimes.com/2005/06/19/magazine/healthconscious.html?_r=0.

1. The Editorial Team, "Forcing Black Men Out of Society," *New York Times*, April 25, 2015, http://www.nytimes.com/2015/04/26/opinion/sunday/forcing-black-men-out-of-society.html?_r=0.

2. William Julius Williams, *When Work Disappears: The New World of the Urban Poor* (Vintage, 1997).

3. Their experience sounds typical of the suite of discriminatory "redlining" practices that extract wealth from poor minorities as they work toward home ownership.

4. See "Chronic Diseases: The Power to Prevent, the Call to Control," Centers for Disease Control, 2009, http://www.cdc.gov/chronicdisease/resources/publications/aag/chronic.htm accessed 2/23/14.

5. "Chronic Care: Making the Case for Ongoing Care," Robert Wood Johnson Foundation, http://www.rwjf.org/content/dam/farm/reports/reports/2010/rwjf54583.

6. M. E. Northridge, A. Morabia, M. L. Ganz, M. T. Bassett, D. Gemson, H. Andrews, and C. McCord, "Contribution of Smoking to Excess Mortality in Harlem," *American Journal of Epidemiology* 147, no. 3 (1998): 250–58, http://www.ncbi.nlm.nih.gov/pubmed/9482499.

7. Ted Alcorn, "Redefining Public Health in New York City," *Lancet* 379, no. 9831 (2012): 2037–38, DOI: http://dx.doi.org/10.1016/S0140-6736(12)60879-4.

8. Ibid., p. 2038.

9. Christopher Bell, *East Harlem Remembered: Oral Histories of Community and Diversity* (McFarland, 2012).

10. Richard Dobbs, Corinne Sawers, Fraser Thompson, James Manyika, Jonathan Woetzel, Peter Child, Sorcha McKenna, and Angela Spatharou, "How the World Could Better Fight Obesity," *Insights & Publications*, McKinsey Institute, November 2014, http://www.mckinsey.com/Insights/Economic_Studies/How_the_world_could_better_fight_obesity?cid=other-eml-alt-mgi-mck-oth-1411.

11. "Chronic Care: Making the Case for Ongoing Care," Robert Wood Johnson Foundation, 2010, http://www.rwjf.org/content/dam/farm/reports/reports/2010/rwjf54583.

12. Robert D. Putnam, *Bowling Alone: The Collapse and Revival of the American Community* (Touchstone Books by Simon & Schuster, 2001).

13. Robert D. Putnam and Lewis Feldstein, *Better Together: Restoring the American Community* (Simon & Schuster, 2004), p. 291.

14. D. S. Tuot, and C. A. Peralta, "To Screen or Not to Screen: That Is Not (Yet) the Question," *Clinical Journal of the American Society of Nephrology* 10, no. 4 (2015): 541–43, DOI: 10.2215/CJN.02150215.

15. Alan E. Guttmacher, M.D., Francis S. Collins, M.D., Ph.D., and Richard H. Carmona, M.D., M.P.H., "The Family History—More Important than Ever," *New England Journal of Medicine* 351 (2004): 2333–36, DOI: 10.1056/NEJMsb042979.

16. "Too Fat to Fight: Retired Military Leaders Want Junk Food Out of America's Schools," Mission: Readiness, http://cdn.missionreadiness.org/MR_Too_Fat_to _Fight-1.pdf.

17. "The Future of the Public's Health in the 21st Century," Institute of Medicine of the National Academies, November 2002, https://www.iom.edu/~/media/Files /Report%20Files/2002/The-Future-of-the-Publics-Health-in-the-21st-Century /Future%20of%20Publics%20Health%202002%20Report%20Brief.pdf.

18. James Colgrove. *Epidemic City: The Politics of Public Health in New York City* (Russell Sage Foundation, 2011), p. 3.

19. Ichiro Kawachi and Lisa F. Berkman, *Neighborhoods and Health* (Oxford University Press, 2003).

20. This builds upon the work started by Mark S. Granovetter in his essay "The Strength of Weak Ties," *American Journal of Sociology* 78, no. 6 (May 1973): 1360–80.

21. Robert J. Sampson, Stephen W. Raudenbush, and Felton Earls, "Neighborhoods and Violent Crime: A Multilevel Study of Collective Efficacy," *Science* 277, no. 5328 (1997): 918–24, DOI: 10.1126/science.277.5328.918.

22. James Coleman introduced "social capital" and "human capital" in his seminal work, "Social Capital in the Creation of Human Capital," *American Journal of Sociology*, Supplement 94 (1988): S95–S120. Robert Putnam has focused upon the civic virtue component of it through his extensive, more popular, writings, such as *Bowling Alone*. The World Bank has described social capital as "not just the sum of the institutions which underpin a society—it is the glue that holds them together." See Partha Dasgupta and Ismail Serageldin, eds., *Social Capital: A Multifaceted Perspective* (World Bank, 1999), p. 44.

23. Eric Foner, *Gateway to Freedom: The Hidden History of the Underground Railroad* (W. W. Norton, 2015).

24. All quotes from Donya Williams in this chapter are from our interview on March 10, 2014.

25. Obesity is defined at a body mass index (BMI) of 30 or greater.

26. "Food Deserts," United States Department of Agriculture Agricultural Marketing Service, http://apps.ams.usda.gov/fooddeserts/foodDeserts.aspx.

27. "Community Health Profiles," New York City Department of Health and Mental Hygiene, 2006, http://www.nyc.gov/html/doh/downloads/pdf/data/2006chp-303.pdf.

28. "Mayor Bloomberg and Speaker Quinn Announce Green Cart Legislation to

Improve Access to Fresh Fruits and Vegetables in Neighborhoods with Greatest Need," NYC Office of the Mayor, December 18, 2007. Available at http://www.nyc.gov/portal /site/nycgov/menuitem.c0935b9a57bb4ef3daf2f1c701c789a0/index.jsp?pageID =mayor_press_release&catID=1194&doc_name=http%3A%2F%2Fwww.nyc.gov %2Fhtml%2Fom%2Fhtml%2F2007b%2Fpr467-07.html&cc=unused1978&rc =1194&ndi=1.

29. "Penn Medicine Experts Offer Suggestions for Nudging Children toward Healthier Food Choices," Penn Medicine, http://www.uphs.upenn.edu/news/News _Releases/2015/03/food/.

30. Steven Cummins, Ellen Flint, and Stephen A. Matthews, "New Neighborhood Grocery Store Increased Awareness of Food Access but Did Not Alter Dietary Habits or Obesity," *Health Affairs* 33, no. 2 (2014): 283–91, DOI: 10.1377/hlthaff.2013.0512.

31. Kathleen Y. Li, B.S., Ellen K. Cromley, Ph.D., Ashley M. Fox, Ph.D., Carol R. Horowitz, M.D., M.P.H., "Evaluation of the Placement of Mobile Fruit and Vegetable Vendors to Alleviate Food Deserts in New York City," *Preventing Chronic Disease* 11 (2014), DOI: 10.5888/pcd11.140086.

32. This entire section owes a heavy debt to the work of Columbia historian James Colgrove, who has written extensively and comprehensively about the history of public health in New York City, and from whom I have drawn and interpreted selectively. His books and articles give a more nuanced and sophisticated view of the evolution of public health in NYC and nationally. This quote comes from Colgrove, "Reform and Its Discontents: Public Health in New York City during the Great Society," *Journal of Political History* 19, no. 1 (2007): 25. Additional quotes from this source are from pp. 17, 30, and 31.

33. Colin McCord and Harold Freeman. "Excess Mortality in Harlem," *New England Journal of Medicine* 322 (1990): 173–77.

34. James A. Hester, John Auerbach, Debbie I. Chang, Sanne Magnan, and Judith Monroe, "Opportunity Knocks Again for Population Health: Round Two in State Innovation Models," Institute of Medicine of the National Academies (2015), http:// www.iom.edu/~/media/Files/Perspectives-Files/2015/SIMsRound2.pdf.

35. George Rust, M.D., M.P.H., David Satcher, M.D., Ph.D., George Edgar Fryer, Ph.D., Robert S. Levine, M.D., and Daniel S. Blumenthal, M.D., M.P.H., "Triangulating on Success: Innovation, Public Health, Medical Care, and Cause-Specific US Mortality Rates over a Half Century (1950–2000)," *American Journal of Public Health* 100, Suppl 1 (2010): S95–104.

36. W. Brian Arthur, *The Nature of Technology: What It Is and How It Evolves* (Free Press, 2011), p. 37.

Chapter 5. The Value of Being Connected

Epigraph. Ben Hecht, "From Community to Prosperity," in *Investing in What Works for America's Communities*, Federal Reserve Bank of San Francisco and Low Income Investment Fund (2012), p. 196.

1. Fred Cerise, "Gov. Bobby Jindal: Why I Opposed Medicaid Expansion," *Times-Picayune*, July 23, 2013, http://www.nola.com/opinions/index.ssf/2013/07/gov_bobby _jindal_why_i_opposed.html.

2. Shushannah Walshe, "Jindal Says He Won't Implement Obamacare," ABC News, June 29, 2012, http://abcnews.go.com/blogs/politics/2012/06/jindal-says-he-wont -implement-obamacare/.

3. "Obamacare's Medicaid Expansion Is Bad for Louisiana," *Greater Baton Rouge Business Report*, https://www.businessreport.com/article/obamacares-medicaid -expansion-is-bad-for-louisiana.

4. The HITECH act launched as part of Troubled Asset Relief Program, which was signed into law by President George W. Bush in 2008.

5. At the time they had 7 mathematicians, 18 engineers, 7 product managers, and 5–6 clinicians.

6. Ruben Amarasingham, Susan H. Spalding, and Ron J. Anderson, "Disease Conditions Most Frequently Evaluated among the Homeless in Dallas," *Journal of Health Care for the Poor and Underserved* 12, no. 2 (2001): 162–76, DOI: 10.1353/ hpu.2010.0765.

7. Glenn Cohen, Ruben Amarasingham, Anand Shah, Bin Xie, and Bernard Lo, "The Legal and Ethical Concerns That Arise from Using Complex Predictive Analytics in Health Care," *Health Affairs* 33, no. 7 (2014): 1139–47, DOI: 10.1377/hlthaff.2014.0048.

8. Ruben Amarasingham, Billy J. Moore, Ying Tabak, Mark H. Drazner, Christopher A. Clark, and Song Zhang, "An Automated Model to Identify Heart Failure Patients at Risk for 30-day Readmission or Death Using Electronic Medical Record Data," *Medical Care* 48, no. 11 (2010): 981–88, DOI: 10.1097/MLR.0b013e3181ef60d9.

9. Ruben Amarasingham, "Applying Data Analytics and Information Exchange to Improve Care for Patients," *Health Affairs* 34, no. 2 (2012): 1, DOI: 10.1377/hlthaff.2012. 1114.

10. Ruben Amarasingham, Parag C. Patel, Kathleen Toto, Lauren L. Nelson, Timothy S. Swanson, Billy J. Moore, Bin Xie, Song Zhang, Kristin S. Alvarez, Ying Ma, Mark H. Drazner, Usha Kollipara, and Ethan A. Halm, "Allocating Scarce Resources in Real-Time to Reduce Heart Failure Readmissions: A Prospective, Controlled Study," *BMJ Quality Safety* 22 (2013): 998–1005, http://qualitysafety.bmj.com/content/22/12 /998.full.pdf+html.

11. Healthify was co-founded by a Baltimore-based alumnus of Health Leads, the organization started by Rebecca Onie (see part 1).

12. Interview with Kimberly Gerra, February 3, 2015.

13. Interview with Anand Shah, January 23, 2015.

14. Cohen et al., "Legal and Ethical Concerns."

15. Interview with Jay Dunn, February 3, 2015.

16. Ibid.

17. Hamilton Moses III, M.D., David H. M. Matheson, J.D., M.B.A., Sarah Cairns-Smith, Ph.D., Benjamin P. George, M.D., M.P.H., Chase Palisch, M.Phil., and E. Ray

Dorsey, M.D., M.B.A., "The Anatomy of Medical Research: US and International Comparisons," *JAMA* 313, no. 2 (2015): 174–89, quote on p. 174, DOI:10.1001/jama. 2014.15939; Bill Gardner, "The Slowing of US Investment in Medical Research," *Incidental Economist*, January 15, 2015, http://theincidentaleconomist.com/wordpress /the-slowing-of-us-investment-in-medical-research/.

18. In the same article, Farmer states that the concept of "race" itself is at the periphery of modern science, while remaining socially significant: "The idea of race, which is considered to be a biologically insignificant term, has enormous social currency." Paul Farmer, "On Suffering and Structural Violence: A View from Below," *Race/Ethnicity: Multidisciplinary Global Contexts* 3, no. 1 (2009): 11–28, quote on p. 30.

Chapter 6. Blessed Are the Organized

Epigraph. Fitzhugh Mullan, "A Founder of Quality Assessment Encounters a Troubled System Firsthand," *Health Affairs* 20, no 1 (2001): 137–41, DOI: 10.1377/ hlthaff.20.1.137.

1. ISAIAH, W. K. Kellogg Foundation, http://www.wkkf.org/grants/grant/2012/06 /the-healthy-heartlands-initiative-3019454.

2. Sponsored by Kresge, Kellogg, and Blue Cross/Blue Shield Foundation, the event took place on November 11, 2014. All quotes from the event in this chapter were captured that day.

3. For more information about the relationships between these fields, please see Manuel Pastor and Rachel Morello-Frosch, "Integrating Public Health and Community Development to Tackle Neighborhood Distress and Promote Well-Being," *Health Affairs* 33, no. 11 (2014): 1890–96, DOI: 10.1377/hlthaff.2014.0640.

4. More recent work on this includes Raj Chetty and Nathaniel Hendren, "The Impacts of Neighborhoods on Intergenerational Mobility: Childhood Exposure Effects and County-Level Estimates" (2015), National Bureau of Economic Research. More information can be found at http://www.equality-of-opportunity.org/.

5. "Advancing Health Equity in Minnesota: Report to the Legislature," Minnesota Department of Health (2014), http://www.health.state.mn.us/divs/chs/healthequity /ahe_leg_report_020414.pdf.

6. Ibid., p. iii.

7. Ibid., pp. 13–14.

8. Ibid., p. 12.

9. "A New Way to Talk about the Social Determinants of Health," Robert Wood Johnson Foundation (2010), http://www.rwjf.org/content/dam/farm/reports/reports /2010/rwjf63023.

10. "Advancing Health Equity in Minnesota," p. 26.

11. Healthy Heartlands Conference, November 11, 2014.

12. Phillip Cryan, "Strategic Practice for Social Transformation," Strategic Practice Grassroots Policy Project, p. 10, http://www.strategicpractice.org/system/files/isaiah _report.pdf.

13. Interview with Doran Schrantz at Healthy Heartlands event, November 11, 2014.

14. Interview with Jeanne Ayers at Healthy Heartlands event, November 11, 2014.

15. Interview with Marlene Hill at Healthy Heartlands event, November 11, 2014.

16. "Training and Strategy," PICO National Network, August 1, 2008, http://www.piconetwork.org/tools-resources/0002.

17. Jillian Olinger, Michelle Oyakawa, Sarah Mullins, Christy Rogers, Doran Schrantz, Jeanne Ayers, and Dave Mann, "Shining the Light: A Practical Guide to Co-Creating Healthy Communities," ISAIAH and the Kirwan Institute for the Study of Race and Ethnicity, May 2010, p. 11, http://isaiahmn.org/newsite/wp-content/uploads/2012/05/Kirwan-Shining-the-Light-Field-Guide-to-Practical-Communities.pdf.

18. "A New Light Rail Line with Stops in Low-Income Neighborhoods," Robert Wood Johnson Foundation, August 4, 2010, http://www.rwjf.org/content/dam/farm/reports/program_results_reports/2010/rwjf70739.

19. Atul Gawande, "The Hot Spotters: Can We Lower Medical Costs by Giving the Neediest Patients Better Care?" *New Yorker*, January 24, 2011, http://www.newyorker.com/magazine/2011/01/24/the-hot-spotters.

20. The estimate of 50 percent is a suggestive number—a small group accounts for a large fraction, and sometimes 40–50 percent is accurate. For more information about this subset and what we do not currently understand, see Tracy Johnson et al., "For Many Patients Who Use Large Amounts of Health Care Services, the Need Is Intense Yet Temporary," *Health Affairs* 34, no. 8 (2015): 1312–19, DOI: 10.1377/hlthaff.2014.1186.

21. Committee on Health Impact Assessment, Board on Environmental Studies and Toxicology, Division on Earth and Life Studies, and National Research Council, *Improving Health in the United States: The Role of Health Impact Assessment* (National Academies Press, 2011), available at http://www.nap.edu/catalog/13229/improving-health-in-the-united-states-the-role-of-health.

22. R. Quigley, L. den Broeder, P. Furu, A. Bond, B. Cave, and R. Bos, *Health Impact Assessment International Best Practice Principles*, Special Publication Series, no. 5 (2006), p. 1, http:// www.iaia.org/publicdocuments/special-publications/SP5.pdf.

23. Interview with Jeanne Ayers at Healthy Heartlands Conference, November 11, 2014.

24. Bethany Rogerson, Ruth Lindberg, Marjory Givens, and Aaron Wernham, "A Simplified Framework for Incorporating Health into Community Development Initiatives," *Health Affairs* 33, no. 11 (2014): 1939–47, DOI: 10.1377/hlthaff.2014.0632.

25. Interview with Jeanne Ayers at Healthy Heartlands Conference, November 11, 2014.

26. Formerly the Pacific Institute for Community Organizations; now only uses the acronym PICO.

27. Shana F. Sandberg, Clese Erikson, Ross Owen, Katherine D. Vickery, Scott T. Shimotsu, Mark Linzer, Nancy A. Garrett, Kimry A. Johnsrud, Dana M. Soderlund, and Jennifer DeCubellis, "Hennepin Health: A Safety-Net Accountable Care

Organization for the Expanded Medicaid Population," *Health Affairs* 33, no. 11 (2014): 1975–84, quote on p. 1975, DOI: 10.1377/hlthaff.2014.0648.

28. Ibid, p. 1977.

29. Ibid, p. 1978.

30. Interview with Paul Marincel at the Healthy Heartlands event, November 11, 2014. Of note, I have not reviewed this data.

31. Ibid.

32. Interview with Jeanne Ayers at Healthy Heartlands Conference, November 11, 2014.

33. Doran M. Schrantz, "Drawing on Community Organizing to Advance Public Health in Minnesota and Beyond," *Health Affairs* 34, no. 12 (2012): 2799–2800, DOI: 10.1377/hlthaff.2012.1112.

34. Interview with Doran Schrantz at Healthy Heartlands event, November 11, 2014.

Chapter 7. Coach Culture

Epigraph. Eames Foundation Webpage, http://www.eamesfoundation.org/, accessed December 15, 2015.

1. Liz Hamel, Jamie Firth, and Mollyann Brodie, "Kaiser Family Foundation/New York Times/CBS Non-Employed Poll," Henry J. Kaiser Family Foundation, December 11, 2014, http://kff.org/other/poll-finding/kaiser-family-foundationnew-york-timescbs-news-non-employed-poll.

2. Atul Gawande, "Personal Best," *New Yorker*, October 3, 2011.

3. Holly C. Felix, Glen P. Mays, M. Kathryn Stewart, Naomi Cottoms, and Mary Olson, "Medicaid Savings Resulted When Community Health Workers Matched Those with Needs to Home and Community Care," *Health Affairs* 30, no. 7 (2011): 1366–74, DOI: 10.1377/hlthaff.2011.0150.

4. APHA (American Public Health Association), "Support for Community Health Workers to Increase Health Access and to Reduce Health Inequities," 2014, https://www.apha.org/policies-and-advocacy/public-health-policy-statements/policy-database/2014/07/09/14/19/support-for-community-health-workers-to-increase-health-access-and-to-reduce-health-inequities, accessed December 12, 2015.

5. "Why Create a Community HUB and Pathways?" *AHRQ Health Care Innovations Exchange*, https://innovations.ahrq.gov/guide/QuickstartGuide/why_create, accessed December 12, 2015.

6. "Enhancing Motivation for Change in Substance Abuse Treatment," in *Treatment Improvement Protocol (TIP)* Series, no. 35, Center for Substance Abuse Treatment, 1999, http://www.ncbi.nlm.nih.gov/books/NBK64964/.

7. Stephen Rollnick, Ph.D., and William R. Miller, Ph.D., "What Is Motivational Interviewing?" *Behavioural and Cognitive Psychotherapy* 23 (1995): 325–34, http://www.motivationalinterview.net/clinical/whatismi.html.

8. "City Health Works Coach Story—Norma," *Cowbird*, http://cowbird.com/story

/101485/City_Health_Works_Coach_Story__Norma/?collectionid=1164anduiid
=widget-2008950827-101485.

9. Earth Institute, Columbia University, "One Million Community Health Workers,"
Technical Task Force Report, http://1millionhealthworkers.org/files/2013/01/1mCHW
_TechnicalTaskForceReport.pdf.

10. Prabhjot Singh and Jeffrey D. Sachs, "1 Million Community Health Workers in
Sub-Saharan Africa by 2015," *Lancet* 382, no. 9889 (2013): 363–65, DOI: http://dx.doi
.org/10.1016/S0140-6736(12)62002-9.

11. They had the benefit of following community health worker programs in the
neighborhood, such as Air Harlem's asthma and environmentally focused efforts,
and New York Presbyterian's Win for Health initiative, and Health Leads.

12. "Dr. Angela Diaz," Robin Hood Foundation, https://www.robinhood.org/about
/dr-angela-diaz.

13. It was named after a famous Harlem pastor who took a stand against the raging
drug epidemic.

14. "The Oberia D. Dempsey Multi-Service Center," West Harlem Group Assistance,
Inc., http://www.whgainc.org/index.php?option=com_content&view=article&id=78
:the-oberia-d-dempsey-multi-service-center&catid=34:demo-category&Itemid=70.

15. Mamelani Projects, http://www.mamelani.org.za/.

16. "Identifying the Active Ingredient: Promoting Adaptation and Global Exchange
of Innovation," Center for Health Market Innovations, http://healthmarketinnovations
.org/sites/default/files/CHMI_ActiveIngredient.pdf.

17. She contributed to this report: Annette Bernhardt, Siobhán McGrath, and
James DeFilippis, "Unregulated Work in the Global City: Employment and Labor
Law Violations in New York City," *Brennan Center for Justice Report* (2007), https://
www.brennancenter.org/sites/default/files/legacy/d/download_file_49436.pdf.

18. Personal interview, August 24, 2014.

19. Personal interview, August 24, 2014.

20. "City Health Works Coach Story—Evelyn," Cowbird, http://cowbird.com/story
/101482/City_Health_Works_Coach_Story__Evelyn/?collectionid=1164anduiid
=widget-900342813-101482.

21. *Appreciation of a system*: understanding the overall processes involving suppli-
ers, producers, and customers (or recipients) of goods and services; *Knowledge of
variation*: the range and causes of variation in quality, and use of statistical sampling
in measurements; *Theory of knowledge*: the concepts explaining knowledge and the
limits of what can be known; *Knowledge of psychology*: concepts of human nature. See
Morgen Witzel and Malcolm Warner, eds., *The Oxford Handbook of Management
Theorists* (Oxford University Press, 2014), pp. 212–13.

22. See Deming's concept of *Profound knowledge* on pp. 211–12 of Witzel and Warner,
eds., *The Oxford Handbook*.

23. Georgett Roberts, Gabrielle Fonrouge, and Natalie O'Neill, "Theater Calls
Cops on Diabetic Man for Bringing in Strawberries," *New York Post*, March 28, 2014,

http://nypost.com/2014/03/28/theater-calls-cops-on-diabetic-man-with-strawberries/.

24. As a nonprofit organization, it is very aware of community-based organizations that have compromised their integrity and effectiveness by blurring the lines between advocacy and political activity.

25. Jürgen Unützer, M.D., M.P.H., Henry Harbin, M.D., Michael Schoenbaum, Ph.D., and Benjamin Druss, M.D., M.P.H., "The Collaborative Care Model: An Approach for Integrating Physical and Mental Health Care in Medicaid Health Homes," Information Resource Center, http://www.medicaid.gov/State-Resource-Center/Medicaid-State-Technical-Assistance/Health-Homes-Technical-Assistance/Downloads/HH-IRC-Collaborative-5-13.pdf.

26. Average ED visit is $2,000, compared to nearly a tenth less for primary care: Nolan Caldwell et al., " 'How Much Will I Get Charged for This?' Patient Charges for Top Ten Diagnoses in the Emergency Department," PLOS One, http://journals.plos.org/plosone/article?id=10.1371/journal.pone.0055491.

27. "Many primary care services currently delivered by physicians, however, can be provided by less costly personnel. An alternative to making an increased investment in primary care training would be to increase the use of complementary, lower-skilled practitioners. Practices that make greater use of lower-cost practitioners, perhaps in combination with highly skilled physicians, are likely to provide higher returns on the societal investment in physician education." More information available here: Sherry A. Glied, Ashwin Prabhu, and Norman H. Edelman, "The Cost of Primary Care Doctors," The National Bureau of Economic Research Working Paper, no. 14568, http://www.nber.org/papers/w14568.pdf. Quote on p. 19.

28. Donald M. Berwick, Thomas W. Nolan, and John Whittington, "The Triple Aim: Care, Health, and Cost," *Health Affairs* 27, no. 3 (2008): 759–69, DOI: 10.1377/hlthaff.27.3.759, quote on p. 759.

29. Maureen Bisognano, "The Vision and Importance of Measuring the Three-Part Aim: Core Metrics for Better Care, Lower Costs, and Better Health" (presentation at an Institute of Medicine workshop at the Beckman Center of National Academies, Irvine, California, December 5, 2013), http://www.iom.edu/~/media/1E672CBCB21445F4A7A08881163A1FEB.ashx.

30. For a case study, see K. Hacker, R. Mechanic, and P. Santos, "Accountable Care in the Safety Net: A Case Study of the Cambridge Health Alliance," Commonwealth Fund, June 2014 http://www.commonwealthfund.org/~/media/files/publications/case-study/2014/jun/1756_hacker_accountable_care_cambridge_ha_case_study_v2.pdf. For an example of scholarship, see Christina Bielaszka-DuVerney, "Taking Public Health Approaches to Care in Massachusetts," *Health Affairs* 6 (2015): 34. For a toolkit, see "Cambridge Health Alliance Model of Team-Based Care Implementation Guide and Toolkits," Cambridge Health Alliance, http://www.integration.samhsa.gov/workforce/team-members/Cambridge_Health_Alliance_Team-Based_Care_Toolkit.pdf.

31. All comments from Soma Stout in this chapter are from a personal interview conducted April 16, 2014.

32. Hacker et al., "Accountable Care in the Safety Net."

33. Marguerite E. Burns, Alison A. Galbraith, Dennis Ross-Degnan, and Richard B. Balaban, "Feasibility and Evaluation of a Pilot Community Health Worker Intervention to Reduce Hospital Readmissions," *International Journal for Quality in Health Care* 26, no. 4 (2014): 358–65, DOI: 10.1093/intqhc/mzu046.

34. Usually refers to the simultaneous payment, delivery, and cultural transformation of a system from volume to value, from healthcare to health.

35. From an event at Harvard Medical School, Longwood Campus, April 16, 2014.

36. Comment made at the 100M Healthier Lives Summit at CMS Headquarters in Baltimore, Maryland, on May 8, 2015.

Chapter 8. The Center Cannot Hold

Epigraph. Harvey Fineberg, "A Successful and Sustainable Health System—How to Get There from Here," *New England Journal of Medicine* 366 (2012): 1024.

1. Personal interview on February 24, 2014, at RWJF media training event in Washington, DC.

2. K. Hacker, R. Mechanic, and P. Santos, "Accountable Care in the Safety Net: A Case Study of the Cambridge Health Alliance," The Commonwealth Fund, June 2014 http://www.commonwealthfund.org/~/media/files/publications/case-study/2014 /jun/1756_hacker_accountable_care_cambridge_ha_case_study_v2.pdf.

3. Bob Herman, "Neighborhood Health Plan Batters Partners HealthCare's Finances in 2014," *Modern Healthcare*, December 12, 2014, http://www.modernhealthcare.com /article/20141212/NEWS/312129959/neighborhood-health-plan-batters-partners -healthcares-finances-in-2014.

4. Mark W. Friedberg, M.D., M.P.P., Eric C. Schneider, M.D., M.Sc., Meredith B. Rosenthal, Ph.D., Kevin G. Volpp, M.D., Ph.D., and Rachel M. Werner, M.D., Ph.D., "Association between Participation in a Multipayer Medical Home Intervention and Changes in Quality, Utilization, and Costs of Care," *JAMA* 311, no. 8 (2014): 815–25, DOI:10.1001/jama.2014.353.

5. Sherry Jacobson, "Top Parkland Managers Won't Get Bonuses for the Last Quarter of 2014," *Dallas Morning News*, April 7, 2015, http://www.dallasnews.com /news/metro/20150407-top-parkland-managers-wont-get-bonuses-for-the-last -quarter-of-2014.ece.

6. Allan Crimm and Don Liss, "Patient-Centered Medical Home Evaluations: Let's Keep Them All in Context," Healthaffairs Blog, May 21, 2014.

7. Kangovi, Shreya, M.D., David Grande, M.D., M.P.A., and Chau Trinh-Shevrin, Dr.P.H., "From Rhetoric to Reality—Community Health Workers in Post-Reform U.S. Health Care," *New England Journal of Medicine* 372 (2015): 2277–79, DOI: 10.1056/ NEJMp1502569.

8. "Integra *ServiceConnect* Adds Some of the Nation's Largest Health Plan Customers in Four States: Unique Service Model Supports Underserved Members in Their Own Communities," *Business Wire*, February 23, 2015, http://www.businesswire.com

/news/home/20150223006155/en/Integra-ServiceConnect-adds-Nations-Largest-Health-Plan#.VU_OQdNViko.

9. Deborah Bachrach, H. Pfister, K. Wallis, and M. Lipson, "Addressing Patients' Social Needs: An Emerging Business Case for Provider Investment," The Commonwealth Fund, May 2014, http://www.commonwealthfund.org/publications/fund-reports/2014/may/addressing-patients-social-needs.

10. Mary Pittman, Anne Sunderland, Andrew Broderick, and Kevin Barnett, "Bringing Community Health Workers into the Mainstream of U.S. Health Care," discussion paper presented at the Roundtable on Population Health Improvement at the Institute of Medicine of the National Academies, February 4, 2015, http://nam.edu/perspectives-2015-bringing-community-health-workers-into-the-mainstream-of-u-s-health-care-2/.

11. "Community Health Workers in California: Sharpening Our Focus on Strategies to Expand Engagement," California Health Workforce Alliance, January 2015, http://www.phi.org/uploads/application/files/2rapr38zarzdgvycgqnizf7o8ftv03ie3mdnioede1ou6s1cv3.pdf.

12. Prabhjot Singh, M.D., Ph.D., and Dave A. Chokshi, M.D., "Community Health Workers—A Local Solution to a Global Problem," *New England Journal of Medicine* 369 (2013): 894–96, DOI: 10.1056/NEJMp1305636.

13. "State Innovation Models Initiative: General Information," Centers for Medicare and Medicaid Services, http://innovation.cms.gov/initiatives/state-innovations/.

14. "Medicaid Expansion in Indiana," Henry J. Kaiser Family Foundation, February 3, 2015, http://kff.org/medicaid/fact-sheet/medicaid-expansion-in-indiana/.

15. "Where the States Stand on Medicaid Expansion: 28 States, D.C. Expanding Medicaid," The Advisory Board Company, February 11, 2015, http://www.advisory.com/daily-briefing/resources/primers/medicaidmap.

16. "Delivery System Transformation Initiatives Proposal for the Massachusetts Section 1115 Waiver: Demonstration Years 15–17," Cambridge Health Alliance, http://www.medicaid.gov/Medicaid-CHIP-Program-Information/By-Topics/Waivers/1115/downloads/ma/MassHealth/ma-masshealth-cambridge-health-dsti-06192012.pdf.

17. "Delivery System Transformation Initiatives (DSTI)," Patient Centered Primary Care Collaborative, webpage accessed December 12, 2015, https://www.pcpcc.org/initiative/delivery-system-transformation-initiatives-dsti.

18. "Where the States Stand on Medicaid Expansion."

19. "Best Care at Lower Cost: The Path to Continuously Learning Health Care in America," Institute of Medicine of the National Academies, http://www.iom.edu/Reports/2012/Best-Care-at-Lower-Cost-The-Path-to-Continuously-Learning-Health-Care-in-America.aspx.

20. "Delivery System Reform Incentive Payment (DSRIP) Program," New York State Department of Health, https://www.health.ny.gov/health_care/medicaid/redesign/dsrip/.

21. Kenneth L. Davis, "Hospital Mergers Can Lower Costs and Improve Medical Care," *Wall Street Journal*, September 15, 2014, http://www.wsj.com/articles/kenneth-l-davis-hospital-mergers-can-lower-costs-and-improve-medical-care-1410823048.

22. Prabhjot Singh and Stuart Butler, "Intermediaries in Integrated Approaches to Health and Economic Mobility," *Economic Studies at Brookings*, No. 4, November 2015.

23. Dan Goldberg, "New York's Leading Health Systems Differ on Growth Strategy," *Capital*, February 9, 2015, http://www.capitalnewyork.com/article/city-hall/2015/02/8561072/new-yorks-leading-health-systems-differ-growth-strategy.

24. Kevin Munjal, M.D., M.P.H., and Brendan Carr, M.D., M.S., "Realigning Reimbursement Policy and Financial Incentives to Support Patient-Centered Out-of-Hospital Care," *JAMA* 309.7 (2013): 667–68, DOI:10.1001/jama.2012.211273.

25. "ONC Market R&D Pilot Challenge," ONC Pilot Challenge, http://www.oncpilotchallenge.com/.

26. Chris DeMars, "Oregon Bridges the Gap between Health Care and Community-Based Health," *Health Affairs Blog*, February 12, 2015, http://healthaffairs.org/blog/2015/02/12/oregon-bridges-the-gap-between-health-care-and-community-based-health/.

27. Icahn School of Medicine at Mount Sinai, "Bundled Payment for Mobile Acute Care Team Services," Centers for Medicare and Medicaid Services, http://innovation.cms.gov/initiatives/Participant/Health-Care-Innovation-Awards-Round-Two/Icahn-School-Of-Medicine-At-Mount-Sinai.html.

28. "Leadership Toolkit for Redefining the H: Engaging Trustees and Communities," American Hospital Association, http://www.aha.org/research/cor/redefiningH/index.shtml?utm_source=newsletterandutm_medium=emailandutm_campaign=NewsNow.

29. James A. Hester and Paul V. Stange, "A Sustainable Financial Model for Community Health Systems" (paper presented during the Institute of Medicine of the National Academies Roundtable on Population Health Improvement, March 2014), http://nam.edu/perspectives-2014-a-sustainable-financial-model-for-community-health-systems/.

30. Sometimes even when public health statistics improve within a community it still feels like it is unhealthy and stagnating, and vice versa. This is analogous to getting great individual-level service and poor healthcare, a concept that increasingly makes less sense.

31. "Integrator Role and Functions in Population Health Improvement Initiatives," Improving Population Health, May 2, 2012, http://www.improvingpopulationhealth.org/Integrator%20role%20and%20functions_FINAL.pdf.

32. This was independent of my involvement with Mount Sinai.

33. David Stark, *The Sense of Dissonance: Accounts of Worth in Economic Life* (Princeton University Press, 2011), p. 15.

34. Mark W. Maier, *The Art of Systems Architecting*, 3rd ed. (CRC Press, 2009).

Chapter 9. From Organizations to Integrators

Epigraph. Nicholas Christakis, quoted in Jonathan Rowson, Steve Broome, and Alasdair Jones, "Connected Communities: How Social Networks Power and Sustain the Big Society," RSA Projects (September 2010), p. 3.

1. Scott Bronstein and Drew Griffin, "A Fatal Wait: Veterans Languish and Die on a VA Hospital's Secret List," CNN, April 24, 2014, http://www.cnn.com/2014/04/23/health/veterans-dying-health-care-delays.

2. Jim Kuhnhenn, "VA Review Finds 'Significant and Chronic' Failures," AP, June 27, 2014, http://bigstory.ap.org/article/obama-hear-update-veterans-affairs-problems.

3. Ashish K. Jha, M.D., Jonathan B. Perlin, M.D., Ph.D., Kenneth W. Kizer, M.D., M.P.H., and R. Adams Dudley, M.D., M.B.A., "Effect of the Transformation of the Veterans Affairs Health Care System on the Quality of Care," *New England Journal of Medicine* 348 (2003): 2218–27, DOI: 10.1056/NEJMsa021899.

4. Telephone interview with Douglas Jutte and David Erickson, February 27, 2015.

5. "$22 Million UnitedHealth Group Investment Helps Fund Three New Affordable-Housing Communities in New Mexico," UnitedHealth Group, June 25, 2013, http://www.unitedhealthgroup.com/newsroom/articles/feed/unitedhealth%20group/2013/0625affordablehousingnewmexico.aspx.

6. Kelly M. Doran, M.D., M.H.S., Elizabeth J. Misa, M.P.A., and Nirav R. Shah, M.D., M.P.H., "Housing as Health Care—New York's Boundary-Crossing Experiment," *New England Journal of Medicine* 369 (2013): 2374–77, DOI: 10.1056/NEJMp1310121.

7. The IOM officially changed its name to the National Academy of Medicine in April 2015. However, for the sake of consistency and recognition, I will continue to use IOM in this book. More information is available at "Press Release: Institute of Medicine to Become National Academy of Medicine," Institute of Medicine of the National Academies, April 28, 2015, http://www.iom.edu/Global/News%20Announcements/IOM-to-become-NAM-Press-Release.aspx.

8. Gardiner Harris, "Vaccine Cleared Again as Autism Culprit," *New York Times*, August 25, 2011.

9. Mary Pittman, Anne Sunderland, Andrew Broderick, and Kevin Barnett, "Bringing Community Health Workers into the Mainstream of U.S. Healthcare," NAM Discussion Paper, February 4, 2015, http://nam.edu/perspectives-2015-bringing-community-health-workers-into-the-mainstream-of-u-s-health-care-2/.

10. *Vital Signs: Core Metrics for Health and Health Care Progress*, IOM Report Website, accessed December 12, 2015, http://iom.nationalacademies.org/Reports/2015/Vital-Signs-Core-Metrics.aspx.

11. Janet Corrigan, Ph.D., M.B.A., Elliott Fisher, M.D., M.P.H., and Scott Heiser, M.P.H., "Hospital Community Benefit Programs Increasing Benefits to Communities," *JAMA* 313, no. 12 (2015): 1211–12, DOI:10.1001/jama.2015.0609.

12. Elliott S. Fisher, M.D., M.P.H., and Janet Corrigan, Ph.D., "Accountable Health Communities: Getting There from Here," *JAMA* 312, no. 20 (2014): 2093–94, DOI: 10.1001/jama.2014.13815.

13. "National Public Health Week," Institute for Health Improvement, April 2015, http://www.ihi.org/Engage/Initiatives/100MillionHealthierLives/Pages /NationalPublicHealthWeek.aspx.

14. "Beyond Health Care: New Directions to a Healthier America," Robert Wood Johnson Foundation, http://www.rwjf.org/content/dam/farm/reports/reports/2009 /rwjf40483.

15. "Time to Act: Investing in the Health of Our Children and Communities," Robert Wood Johnson Foundation, http://www.rwjf.org/content/dam/farm/reports /reports/2014/rwjf409002.

16. Risa Lavizzo-Mourey, "Building a Culture of Health," Robert Wood Johnson Foundation, http://www.rwjf.org/en/library/annual-reports/presidents-message -2014.html.

17. E. E. Kersten, K. Z. LeWinn, L. Gottlieb, D. P. Jutte, and N. E. Adler, "San Francisco Children Living in Redeveloped Public Housing Used Acute Services Less than Children in Older Public Housing," *Health Affairs* 33, no. 12 (2014): 2230–37, DOI: 10.1377/ hlthaff.2014.1021.

18. Maggie Super Church, "Neighborhood Health: A New Framework for Investing in Sustainable Communities," *Community Development Investment Review*, March 2014, http://www.frbsf.org/community-development/files/cdir_vol10issue1-Neighborhood -Health.pdf.

19. "HHS FY2015 Budget in Brief," U.S. Department of Health and Human Services, http://www.hhs.gov/about/budget/fy2015/budget-in-brief/index.html.

20. Laura R. Wherry, Sarah Miller, Robert Kaestner, and Bruce D. Meyer, "Childhood Medicaid Coverage and Later Life Health Care Utilization," National Bureau of Economic Research, Working Paper No. 20929, February 2015, DOI: 10.3386/w20929.

21. Karen Eggleston and Victor R. Fuchs, "The New Demographic Transition: Most Gains in Life Expectancy Now Realized Late in Life," Working Paper Series No. 29, Asian Health Policy Program, the Walter H. Shorenstein Asia-Pacific Research Center, Stanford University, http://iis-db.stanford.edu/pubs/23743/AHPPwp_29.pdf.

22. "Do Retirees Receive More from Medicare than They Pay In?" Harvard School of Public Health/SSRS Poll, May 13–26, 2013, http://cdn1.sph.harvard.edu/wp-content /uploads/sites/21/2013/09/HSPH-Medicare-charts.pdf.

23. Personal interview with Peggy Honoré, January 15, 2015.

24. James J. Heckman and Stefano Mosso, "The Economics of Human Development and Social Mobility," National Bureau of Economic Research, Working Paper No. 19925, February 2014, DOI: 10.3386/w19925.

25. Janet M. Corrigan, Ph.D., and Elliott S. Fisher, M.D., M.P.H., "Accountable Health Communities: Insights from State Health Reform Initiatives," Current FAQs, Dartmouth Institute for Health Policy and Clinical Practice, November 2014, http:// tdi.dartmouth.edu/images/uploads/AccountHealthComm-WhPaperFinal.pdf.

26. Personal communication, David Erickson.

27. "What Are the Federal Reserve's Objectives in Conducting Monetary Policy?"

Board of Governors of the Federal Reserve System, http://www.federalreserve.gov
/faqs/money_12848.htm.

28. Primary Care Development Corporation, available at http://www.pcdc.org
/about-us/our-impact.html.

29. *Investing in What Works for America's Communities: Essays on People, Place, and
Purpose,* Nancy Andrews and David Erickson, senior editors (Federal Reserve Bank of
San Francisco and Low Income Investment Fund, 2012) and *What Counts: Harnessing
Data for America's Communities,* Naomi Cytron, Kathryn L. S. Pettit, and G. Thomas
Kingsley, senior editors (Federal Reserve Bank of San Francisco and the Urban Insti-
tute, 2014).

30. The number 200,000 is rough and can be derived from the definition of a
"block group" in the 2010 census, which is available at "2010 Census Tallies of Census
Tracts, Block Groups & Blocks," United States Census Bureau, https://www.census.gov
/geo/maps-data/data/tallies/tractblock.html.

31. 100 Million Healthier Lives Overview, webpage, http://www.ihi.org/Engage
/Initiatives/100MillionHealthierLives/Pages/default.aspx, accessed December 13, 2015.

Chapter 10. SCALE at the Speed of Relationships

Epigraph. *Investing in What Works for America's Communities: Essays on People, Place,
and Purpose,* Nancy Andrews and David Erickson, senior editors (Federal Reserve
Bank of San Francisco and Low Income Investment Fund, 2012), p. 378.

1. James J. Heckman and Stefano Mosso, "The Economics of Human Development
and Social Mobility," National Bureau of Economic Research, Working Paper No.
19925, February 2014, DOI: 10.3386/w19925.

2. Intelligent Collaborative Knowledge Networks, http://www.ickn.org.

3. "Collaborative Improvement and Innovation Network to Reduce Infant Mortality (IM CoIIN)," NICHQ, http://www.nichq.org/childrens-health/infant-health/coiin
-to-reduce-infant-mortality.

4. Peter A. Gloor, Carey Heckmann, and Fillia Makedon, "Ethical Issues in Collaborative Innovation Networks," Online Working Paper, accessed December 13, 2015,
http://www.ickn.org/documents/COIN4Ethicomp.pdf.

5. "Robert Wood Johnson Foundation Awards IHI $4.8 Million to Help Communi-
ties Become National and Global Models of Health," Robert Wood Johnson Foundation, http://www.rwjf.org/en/about-rwjf/newsroom/newsroom-content/2015/01
/robert-wood-johnson-foundation-awards-ihi--4-8-million-to-help-c.html.

6. Elinor Ostrom, "Green from the Grassroots," Project Syndicate, June 12, 2012,
http://www.project-syndicate.org/commentary/green-from-the-grassroots.

7. Elinor Ostrom, "Beyond Markets and States: Polycentric Governance of Complex Economic Systems," *American Economic Review* 100 (2010): 1–33, http://bnp
.binghamton.edu/wp-content/uploads/2011/06/Ostrom-2010-Polycentric
-Governance.pdf.

8. John Kania and Mark Kramer, "Collective Impact," *Stanford Social Innovation*

Review (Winter 2011), http://www.ssireview.org/articles/entry/collective_impact.

9. Janet Corrigan, Ph.D., M.B.A., Elliott Fisher, M.D., M.P.H., and Scott Heiser, M.P.H., "Hospital Community Benefit Programs Increasing Benefits to Communities," *JAMA* 313, no.12 (2015): 1211–12, DOI:10.1001/jama.2015.0609.

10. "Robert Wood Johnson Foundation Launches Initiative to Assess How Data Can Be Used to Improve Health," Robert Wood Johnson Foundation, October 16, 2014, http://www.rwjf.org/en/library/articles-and-news/2014/10/RWJFLaunchesInitiative toAccessHowDataCanBeUsedtoImproveHealth.html. See also "A Robust Health Data Infrastructure," Agency for Healthcare Research and Quality, Publication No. 14-0041-EF, April 2014 http://healthit.gov/sites/default/files/ptp13-700hhs_white.pdf.

11. "Open Notes," Robert Wood Johnson Foundation, http://www.rwjf.org/en /how-we-work/grants/grantees/OpenNotes.html.

12. "Defining Small Data," Small Data Group, October 18, 2013, http:// smalldatagroup.com/2013/10/18/defining-small-data.

13. "What's Possible with Open mHealth?" Open mHealth, http://www .openmhealth.org/features/features-overview.

14. Telephone interview with Deborah Estrin, March 6, 2015.

15. Committee on Networked Systems of Embedded Computers, Computer Science and Telecommunications Board, Division on Engineering and Physical Sciences, and National Research Council, *Embedded, Everywhere: A Research Agenda for Networked Systems of Embedded Computers* (National Academy Press, 2001). Available at http:// www.nap.edu/openbook.php?record_id=10193.

16. Telephone interview with Douglas Jutte and David Erickson, February 27, 2015.

17. "On Consensus and Humming in the IETF," Internet Engineering Task Force, https://tools.ietf.org/html/draft-resnick-on-consensus-00#page-10.

18. "IHI Announces Final Selection of Communities for Health-Focused SCALE Initiative," Institute for Healthcare Improvement, April 17, 2015, http://www.ihi.org /about/news/Documents/IHIPressRelease_IHIAnnouncesSCALEAwardees_Apr15.pdf.

Chapter 11. Integrating the Whole

Epigraph. David Cutler, *The Quality Cure: How Focusing on Health Care Quality Can Save Your Life and Lower Spending Too* (University of California Press, 2014), p. 90.

1. Theodore R. R. Marmor, Morris L. Barer, and Robert G. Evans, eds., *Why Are Some People Healthy and Others Not? The Determinants of Health Populations* (Aldine Transaction, 1994), p. 29.

2. David Kindig and Greg Stoddart, "What Is Population Health?" *American Journal of Public Health* 93, no. 3 (2003): 380–83, DOI: 10.2105/AJPH.93.3.380.

3. Dawn Marie Jacobson, M.D., M.P.H., and Steven Teutsch, M.D., M.P.H., "An Environmental Scan of Integrated Approaches for Defining and Measuring Total Population Health by the Clinical Care System, the Government Public Health System, and Stakeholder Organizations," Improving Population Health, http:// www.improvingpopulationhealth.org/PopHealthPhaseIICommissionedPaper.pdf.

4. Committee on Quality Measures for the Healthy People Leading Health Indica-tors, Board on Population Health and Health Practice, and Institute of Medicine, *Toward Quality Measures for Population Health and the Leading Health Indicators* (National Academies Press, 2013).

5. Benjamin L. Howell, Ph.D., Patrick H. Conway, M.D., and Rahul Rajkumar, M.D., "Guiding Principles for Center for Medicare & Medicaid Innovation Model Evaluations," *JAMA* 313, no. 23 (2015): 2317–18, DOI:10.1001/jama.2015.2902.

6. Raj Chetty, Nathaniel Hendren, and Lawrence Katz, "The Effects of Exposure to Better Neighborhoods on Children: New Evidence from the Moving to Opportunity Experiment," Equality of Opportunity, May 2015, http://www.equality-of -opportunity.org/images/mto_exec_summary.pdf.

7. Linda T. Kohn, Janet M. Corrigan, and Molla S. Donaldson, eds., *To Err Is Human: Building a Safer Health System* (National Academies Press, 2000).

8. Peggy A. Honoré, Donald Wright, Donald M. Berwick, Carolyn M. Clancy, Peter Lee, Juleigh Nowinski, and Howard K. Koh, "Creating a Framework for Getting Quality into the Public Health System," *Health Affairs* 30, no. 4 (2011): 737–45, DOI: 10.1377/hlthaff.2011.0129.

9. Elizabeth A. McGlynn, Ph.D., and John L. Adams, Ph.D., "What Makes a Good Quality Measure?" *JAMA* 312, no. 15 (2014): 1517–18, DOI:10.1001/jama.2014.12819.

10. "Accountability—The Pathway for Restoring Public Trust and Confidence for Hospitals and Other Health Care Organizations," American Hospital Association, Working Paper, November 1999, accessed December 12, 2015, http://www.aha.org /content/00-10/AHAPrinciplesAccountability.pdf.

11. L. D. Gamm, "Dimensions of Accountability for Not-for-Profit Hospitals and Health Systems," *Health Care Management Review* 21, no. 2 (1996): 74–86.

12. Ezekiel J. Emanuel, M.D., Ph.D., and Linda L. Emanuel, M.D., Ph.D., "What Is Accountability in Health Care?" *Annals of Internal Medicine* 124 (2006): 229–39, http:// services.medicine.uab.edu/PublicDocuments/Anesthesiology/JC0414Art2.pdf.

13. Total per capita costs for everyone in a neighborhood (a total population) is not readily available, for a myriad of reasons, although it is knowable with significant effort. It is difficult enough to know the total per capita costs for a well-defined subpopulation if multiple insurers are involved. For specific references to drug prices, see Peter Loftus, "How Much Should Cancer Drugs Cost?" *Wall Street Journal*, June 18, 2015, http://www.wsj.com/articles/how-much-should-cancer-drugs-cost -1434640914. For references to insurance premiums, see Avery Johnson, "Expect Health-Insurance Premiums to Rise," *Wall Street Journal*, March 22, 2014, http://www .wsj.com/articles/SB10001424052702304756104579449153495552222. For comments on overall healthcare costs, see Drew Altman, "New Evidence Health Spending Is Growing Faster Again," *Washington Wire*, June 11, 2015, http://blogs.wsj.com/washwire /2015/06/11/new-evidence-health-spending-is-growing-faster-again.

14. Tyler Norris, "Total Health: Public Health and Health Care in Action," Total

Health Partnerships, Kaiser Permanente, http://healthyamericans.org/assets/files /TFAH2013HealthierAmericaXrpt03.pdf, accessed December 13, 2015.

15. All quotes in this chapter from Peggy Honoré are from a personal interview, January 15, 2015.

16. Russel Honoré is a distant relation who played an instrumental role in the post-Katrina response; the professorship was chosen by LSU independent of this coincidental relationship. Peggy Honoré teaches at Tulane, University of Southern Mississippi, Medical University of South Carolina, and George Washington University.

17. Peggy A. Honoré, et al., "Creating a Framework for Getting Quality into the Public Health System."

18. Institute of Medicine, *For the Public's Health: The Role of Measurement in Action and Accountability* (National Academies Press, 2011), p. 5, http://iom.nationalacademies .org/Reports/2010/For-the-Publics-Health-The-Role-of-Measurement-in-Action-and -Accountability.aspx.

19. Gustavo Solis, "Group Calls for Moratorium on New Drug-Related Programs in East Harlem," *DNAinfo New York*, June 23, 2015, http://www.dnainfo.com/new-york /20150504/east-harlem/group-calls-for-moratorium-on-new-drug-related-programs -east-harlem.

Chapter 12. Imagining the Future Out Loud

Epigraph. Arthur Kleinman, "Caregiving as Moral Experience," *Lancet* 380, no. 9853 (November 2012): 1550–51, http://dx.doi.org/10.1016/S0140-6736(12)61870-4.

1. "Better, Smarter, Healthier: In Historic Announcement, HHS Sets Clear Goals and Timeline for Shifting Medicare Reimbursements from Volume to Value," US Department of Health and Human Services, January 26, 2015, http://www.hhs.gov /news/press/2015pres/01/20150126a.html.

2. Corita Grudzen, Lynne D. Richardson, Kevin M. Baumlin, Gary Winkel, Carine Davila, Kristen Ng, Ula Hwang, and the GEDI WISE Investigators, "Redesigned Geriatric Emergency Care May Have Helped Reduce Admissions of Older Adults to Intensive Care Units," *Health Affairs* 34, no. 5 (2015): 788–95, DOI: 10.1377/hlthaff.2014.0790.

3. "Emerging Positions in Primary Care: Results from the 2014 Ambulatory Care Workforce Survey," Greater New York Hospital Association, http://nyachnyc.org/wp -content/uploads/2015/04/GNYHAAmbulatoryCareReport_compress.pdf.

4. Spotlight 1199SEIU Funds, May 2015, https://www.1199seiubenefits.org/wp -content/uploads/2015/05/May-1-2015-League.html.

5. For more detail, see Prabhjot Singh and Stuart M. Butler, "Intermediaries in Integrated Approaches to Health and Economic Mobility," Economic Studies at Brookings, No. 4, November 2015, http://www.brookings.edu/~/media/research/files /papers/2015/11/30-intermediaries-in-integrated-approaches-to-health-and -economic-mobility-singh-butler/intermediaries_in_integrated_approaches_to _health_and_econ_mobility.pdf.

6. João Biehl and Adriana Petrenya, eds., *When People Come First: Critical Studies in Global Health* (Princeton University Press, 2013).

7. "Life Expectancy Map," Robert Wood Johnson Foundation, http://www.rwjf.org /en/library/infographics/life-expectancy-map--new-york-city.html.

8. Robert D. Putnam, "Lonely in America," *Atlantic Online*, September 21, 2000, https://www.theatlantic.com/past/docs/unbound/interviews/ba2000-09-21.htm.

9. "Public Lives: A Budget Wizard Trades His Wand for a Tourniquet," *New York Times*, February 12, 2002, http://www.nytimes.com/2002/02/12/nyregion/public-lives -a-budget-wizard-trades-his-wand-for-a-tourniquet.html.

10. W. Brian Arthur, "Increasing Returns and the New World of Business," *Harvard Business Review* 75, no. 4 (July-August 1996), https://hbr.org/1996/07/increasing -returns-and-the-new-world-of-business.

11. Rita Gunther McGrath and Ian MacMillan, "Discovery-Driven Planning," *Harvard Business Review*, 73, no. 4 (July 1995): 44–54. For the reintroduced concept, see Rita Gunther McGrath and Ian MacMillan, *Discovery-Driven Growth: A Breakthrough Process to Reduce Risk and Seize Opportunity* (Harvard Business Review Press, 2009).

12. Prabhjot Singh. "Tomorrow's Health Relies on New Relationships," *Stanford Social Innovation Review*, June 24, 2015, http://www.ssireview.org/blog/entry /tomorrows_health_relies_on_new_relationships.

13. In fact, one of Sanghavi's other projects at CMMI, aside from the AHC, is the Million Hearts initiative to prevent 1 million heart attacks by 2017.

14. W. Brian Arthur, *The Nature of Technology: What It Is and How It Evolves* (Free Press, 2011).

Index

1:1 interactions: in confronting tensions, 132; in organizing, 115, 117–19, 124, 128–29, 130
10-point health plan (Young Lords), 81–83
100 Million Healthier Lives (100M) Campaign, 168–71, 178–81, 202–5, 212–16; rough consensus in, 214–16, 239; SCALE in, 185, 197–201; Summit, 176–77

ACA (Patient Protection and Affordable Care Act), 2–3, 38–39, 43–47, 97–98, 233
accountability, 211–12, 227–28, 234–37, 238, 241–42
ACO (accountable care organization), 44–45, 149, 151
activism, 115, 122–23, 124, 190
adaptive problem solving: coaches in, 147–48; communications in, 106–7; confronting tensions in, 115–16, 129; IEP in, 105; leadership in, 106, 129, 132; local pioneers in, 91–92; technical/community approach to, 92, 120–24
"Advancing Health Equity in Minnesota" (Minnesota Department of Health), 111–16
advocacy/advocates, 120, 127, 136, 147
African Americans, 55, 56, 59–60, 110, 111
AHA (American Hospital Association), 164, 227
AHC (Accountable Health Community), 183, 191, 192, 204, 222–23, 236
AIC (Academic Innovations Collaborative), 153–54
alliances, 44, 114–15, 248
alternative sources of healthcare, 237–38
Amarasingham, Ruben, 91–92, 95–97, 102
"America's Health in Transition" (IOM), 233–34
analytics, 94–95, 100, 103, 206
Anderson, Ron, 93–95, 98
Antonovsky, Aaron, 52
APHA (American Public Health Association), 135–36, 183–84
Arrow, Kenneth J., 39–40
Arthur, W. Brian, 86, 249, 251–52
austerity, narratives of, 119, 120, 123
Ayers, Jean, 111, 115–17, 119–20, 122, 123, 124, 131

behavior, 30, 31, 70–72, 77–79, 229
behavioral health, 104, 149, 236
Berwick, Don, 37, 148
Beyond Majority Rules: Voteless Decisions in the Religious Society of Friends, 215–16
biomedical research, 5–6, 19, 20, 181
birth-to-college services, 63–64
Bloomberg, Michael, 75–77
Blue Zone Project, 67–68
bodegas, 76–78, 236–37
Brenner, Jeffrey, "The Hotspotters," 121
Bridge, the, 104
Brill, Steven, "The Bitter Pill," 41–42
Brown, Howard J., 80–81
Build Healthy Places Network, 186–87
business development, 62–63, 99

Canada, Geoffrey, 63
care coordination/coordinators, 103, 134–35, 145–46, 150
caregivers/caregiving, 72, 241
Carmona, Rob, 217–18, 243
CDC (Centers for Disease Control), 75, 183, 188
CDCs (community development corporations), 58, 192–93
CDFIs (community development financing institutions), 58–59, 162, 178–79, 194
Cerise, Fred, 92–95, 103–4
CHA (Cambridge Health Alliance), 149–54, 156, 159–60, 216
change, theories of, 204–5, 208–9
change leaders/agents, 147–48, 151, 176, 180–81, 194–95. *See also* pioneers
charge masters, 41
CHC (community health centers), 24, 222–23
"cheap talk": in DSRIP, 162; in future Harlem, 243, 246, 248; in Healthy Heartlands, 111; on neighborhood issues, 65–66; pathways for, 239; in rough consensus, 216; in SCALE, 201; in systems development, 86; value of, 106–7
childhood development, 184–85, 186, 190–91, 251
children's health, 186, 188, 190–91, 193
children's programs, 63–64, 140, 184–85, 217

283